# Homeopathy Rising

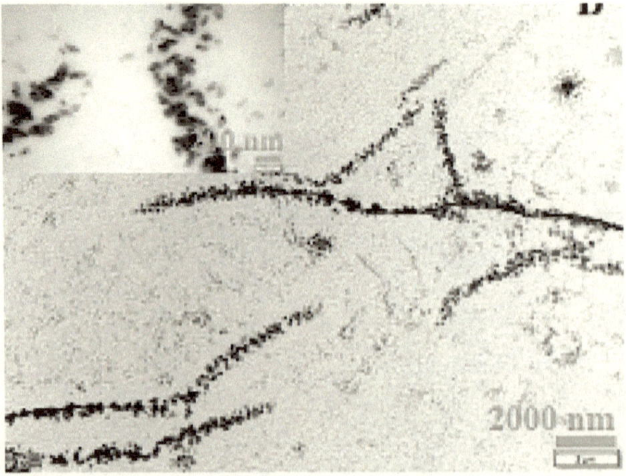


*Transmission electron microscope images of complex nanostructures in a homeopathic remedy solution. Used by permission. Full credits follow the index.*

# Homeopathy Rising

*A Deep Introduction to Earth's Fastest Growing Medicine*

S. Marjorie Ratliff

Twelve Winds Press

Homeopathy Rising: A Deep Introduction to Earth's Fastest Growing Medicine
Twelve Winds Press
twelvewindspress.com

ISBN: 978-1-0691765-2-3


The information and ideas in this book are not medical advice and cannot replace consultation with a qualified healthcare professional.

Due to the passion and perseverance of
research teams worldwide, the door is now
open to more precise scientific study of
homeopathy, and a new era in medicine.
This book is dedicated to them.

Emerging data and new theoretical work are creating a quiet revolution in homeopathy. The evidence is published and accessible.

*Iris Bell, PhD, MD, MD(H)*

Homeopathy is an applied science, not a theory. The sick are entitled to exact knowledge, not to guesswork.

*James Tyler Kent, MD*

Children often resist taking a conventional medicine. Perhaps they are trying to tell us something.

*Dana Ullman, MPH, CCH*

# Contents

A note to the reader

1 What is homeopathy? 1

2 How is it different from conventional medicine? 7

3 Is a homeopath a naturopath or an herbalist? 21

4 Why would I try homeopathic healthcare? 27

5 What is the origin of homeopathy? 39

6 How does it work? 45

7 Is there scientific research on homeopathy? 61

8 Why is homeopathy controversial? 71

9 Is it true that homeopathy is a placebo? 77

10 I tried a remedy and it didn't work. Why? 83

11 How should I choose a homeopath? 89

12 Eight cases 115

13 Food for thought 133

References

Index

# A note to the reader

When I first encountered homeopathy, there was little information for newcomers. Now there is much more. But I felt this book would be welcomed by those who—like me—want to understand something more deeply before jumping in. The details, the big picture; the how and why. It's a book I would have liked to have back then.

This book is arranged to address the most commonly asked questions. Read patiently. Pause often to think and imagine, and expect to revisit. If it's completely new to you, it may seem complicated at first, but truly, classical homeopathy's great power lies in its sound, timeless simplicity. It's from nature that strength and healing come, and nature is wonderfully ordered. Its founder, Dr. Hahnemann, put it this way:

> *The highest ideal of cure is rapid, gentle, and permanent restoration of the health, in the shortest, most reliable, and most harmless way, on easily comprehensible principles.*

Homeopathy offers nothing less than a new way of life. One day you may be amazed that you ever lived without its humanity and wisdom.

# 1
# What is homeopathy?

Homeopathy is a holistic scientific healthcare system which has been meticulously developed over the past 230 years. It is based on timeless laws of the natural world which govern all living organisms, and which have been observed everywhere on Earth for millennia. These laws or principles of life are now being verified by the most advanced scientific research of our time.

This book offers an overview of the principles upon which classical homeopathy was built, and which have sustained its success for more than two centuries. Within it, you will find information and context which can help you make informed choices about your healthcare. Common misconceptions are explained, and some of the fundamentally flawed criticisms of homeopathy's vocal pseudoskeptics are examined.

Some modern practitioners use the homeopathic remedies (the odd little white pills) but do not follow the guiding principles of classical homeopathy. We will look at a few of the most important new methodologies, to help you understand the different types of practice so you can make your own decisions about which is right for you.

Because it is effective, affordable, and gentle to our bodies, hundreds of millions of people around the world choose homeopathic care, making it one of the most commonly used medical systems, according to a 2019 meta-analysis by the World Health Organization (WHO).[1] Homeopathic care is integrated into public health services in many countries, including Switzerland, Brazil, India, Chile, and Mexico, among others. In most places homeopaths are licensed medical doctors who study homeopathy as a medical specialty with extra years of training, just as oncologists, surgeons, and other specialists do.

Thirty percent of European citizens use homeopathy; in countries with the highest rates of health literacy, a majority of people use homeopathy for some or all of their health concerns. In 2023, researchers found that of residents of Germany, Spain, and Italy who had used homeopathy, averaged between the three nations eighty-five percent were satisfied with the outcome.[2] Polls in the United States for the same year found more than seventy percent of Americans said conventional medicine was failing them in several critical respects.[3] Interest in alternative medical systems, including homeopathy, has been growing rapidly in North America for decades. In Canada alone, more than ten million people (about a quarter of the population) said they used homeopathic medicine in 2022.[4] Over forty percent of global spending on homeopathy in 2025 is projected to occur in the United States.[5] Yet it is still widely misunderstood and marginalized.

Throughout its history, homeopathy has been the chosen healthcare of many highly educated people who had access to state-of-the-art conventional medicine. Champions of homeopathy have included figures as diverse as one could imagine: Abraham Lincoln, Charles Darwin, Mahatma Gandhi, Florence Nightingale, Elizabeth Cady Stanton, John D. Rockefeller, Ludwig van Beethoven, the British royal family, Usain Bolt, David Beckham, Mother Theresa, Johann Wolfgang von Goethe, Charles Dickens, Ralph Waldo Emerson, Paul McCartney, Dizzy Gillespie, Tina Turner, Yehudi Menuhin, Mark Twain, Cher, Jude Law, and countless others from all walks of life—from popes to presidents. Entire books have been written about the subject. Nobel laureates Brian Josephson and Luc Montagnier have been among the prominent scientists who put their reputations on the line by advocating for homeopathy.

As you read this book, it will become clear why so many people choose homeopathy. It strengthens our natural immunity and stimulates our innate capacity for healing. When properly used, it does not create side effects. It is appropriate for people at any age, including during pregnancy. It is effective in chronic conditions, epidemics, palliative care, and many first aid or acute situations. Homeopathy is often an ideal option for children's health problems since it is completely non-toxic and non-addictive. It often relieves the need for antibiotics and other medications, and actively supports the development of a robust, efficient immune system.

One reason homeopathy is growing in popularity is that it can help those caught up in the accelerating modern pandemic of autoimmune disorders and the many other inflammatory and degenerative conditions for which conventional medicine offers no real hope. It can be of use for people with conditions such as asthma, allergies, attention disorders, migraines, menstrual and menopause difficulties, sleep disorders, emotional trauma, cognitive challenges, and recurrent infections, to name just a few common problems. With correct management it can be used on its own or combined with other therapies. By increasing our resilience, homeopathic treatment sets us up for a healthier future.

A good homeopath is a highly skilled practitioner with extensive training. They have learned to interpret the human organism's many ways of expressing what kind of help it needs. A long first interview explores any physical signs and sensations, emotions and moods, temperament, mental habits, family and personal health histories. Perceiving all of this information as an integrated whole, and designing an individualized plan for restoring health, is a science and an art.

Homeopathy uses a unique set of medicinal preparations known as *remedies,* which are produced through a strictly regulated process. The specific qualities of hundreds of remedies have been thoroughly explored and documented through lengthy double-blind in vivo studies called *provings.* For more than two hundred years clinical observations have been added to the body of knowledge. Research into the substance and action of the remedies has intensified in recent years, thanks to extremely sensitive new technologies. Paradigm-changing results are emerging from research centers worldwide.

This well loved healthcare system has persisted for centuries in spite of obstinate opposition and bias, lack of funding and educational opportunities, and widespread misinformation. In the twenty-first century its usership is growing exponentially. Mainstream science is now catching up, becoming better equipped to illuminate its processes. If it remains rooted in the natural laws that it was founded on, homeopathy's continued expansion and integration are assured.

# 2
# How is homeopathy different from conventional medicine?

Over the last two centuries, numerous new modalities have sprouted from mainstream medicine. Each has grown in a unique direction; each offers a more nuanced and holistic approach than the conventional model from which it emerged. These modalities include (in order of appearance) homeopathy, osteopathy, and chiropractic.

All of these were founded by medical doctors who recognized that human beings have a powerful, innate potential for healing. They saw that conventional medicine was operating with a very narrow view of sickness and health. Heedless of our natural propensity for healing, it was overpowering the body with drugs (and sometimes unnecessary surgeries), even when gentle, holistic treatments were more appropriate.

These innovations were based on the certainty that medical interventions did not need to be harmful. Their practitioners found that great progress could be made in cases considered incurable by medical doctors when the natural healing process was supported.

In some ways, a consultation with a homeopath is quite similar to seeing a doctor. In both cases, your health history and current condition are assessed (though the homeopath will ask for much more information about your overall health, and will inquire about your individual constitution). Based on your situation, a decision is reached whether any intervention is needed. Once a plan is implemented, the results must be thoughtfully discussed and evaluated periodically. In both scenarios, change may be rapid or may require a patient and careful stepwise strategy.

One fundamental difference between the two is that classical homeopathy is based on a small number of timeless principles or natural laws. Conventional medicine, surprisingly, has no coherent philosophy or principles for understanding what good health is, or how to help bring it about. Definitions such as "health is the absence of pain or disease" or "health is a state of well-being" are too superficial to guide treatment. They do not touch the questions of how or why healing happens. Without sound theory, practice is continually pieced together ad hoc and adjusted painfully when it turns out it has gone wrong. This approach is, at least in part, perpetuated by the manner in which conventional medical drugs are developed.

In classical homeopathy, practice is inseparable from the fundamental theory. Together they are rooted unshakably in the definition of health which life itself offers us, when we're willing and able to observe it with an open mind. The German polymath who founded homeopathy as a medical practice put it this way: when a person is in good health, the vital, animating energy of life sustains

> *...all the parts of the organism in admirable, harmonious, vital operation, as regards both sensations and functions, so that our indwelling, reason-gifted mind can freely employ this living, healthy instrument for the higher purpose of our existence.*

This passage from homeopathy's first, and still most important, text, *Organon of the Medical Art,* expresses the foundational homeopathic view of a human being. Each of us is endowed with a meaningful inner life, and a purpose in the broader context of our community and the world. When we are sick, our freedom, our happiness, and our productivity are restricted. Healing means the restoration, or creation, of that ordered, harmonized functioning so that we can live to our full potential.

By extension—and this is explicit in homeopathy—medicine is for the healing of humanity, not only for isolated people with diagnosed diseases, at particular moments in their lives. The homeopathic world view affirms that healthy people will not enact violence on each other or on the Earth, our home.

In everyday practice, this theoretical strength means that in classical homeopathy there is a consistent and rational basis for observation and action. There is a scale upon which to measure sickness and wellness. Symptoms can be analyzed in the context of the entire organism, and in the context of a complete lifetime. A coherent plan can be designed for increasing strength and resilience. Progress or degeneration can be evaluated rationally, according to an organized understanding of the whole spectrum of health.

Homeopaths recognize that an innate energy in living things not only gives them life, but guides their development, growth, adaptation, and healing. Every seed that germinates, every baby that is born and grows through the stages of life, every illness or injury that heals "by itself" demonstrates this fundamental natural property of living things. Cells and organs, humans and plants and animals, indeed whole ecosystems, do not grow at random; their development is intricately organized. It is invariably oriented toward healing, regeneration, adaptation, and problem-solving.

Traditionally, homeopaths have called this energy of life the *vital force*. Some are now warily avoiding that term (indeed I was advised to remove it from this book) because it has been labeled "unscientific." I will show that it is not in the least unscientific for medicine to acknowledge the self-organizing impulse which governs biological systems. On the contrary, denying the energy which gives us life is not only unscientific but senseless. It is time for the hostile detractors to see their denials for what they are: entrenched emotional habits which obstruct the ability to engage with the true spirit of science, which ultimately is about learning, not about clinging to comfortable but obsolete formulations.

We are endowed with life; we heal every day, or we would not continue to live. Throughout this book, I will refer to the vital energy, vital force, or natural healing process, interchangeably. It is a central concept, because the one and only purpose of a correctly chosen homeopathic remedy is to support and amplify the natural energy of life which is always working in us.

Homeopathy differs from conventional medicine in that it is a *similar* medicine. The remedies are intended to work *with* the natural healing process, rather than against it. This concept will be explored all through this book. It can take some time to comfortably view health, sickness, and medicine through this lens, but it is so worthwhile; it gives a new perspective which extends to other aspects of life. Homeopathy is rooted in a profoundly non-violent and appreciative outlook which benefits ourselves and others.

Conventional medical treatment is almost always *contrary* medicine. Rather than viewing sickness as an experience of the entire person, it tends to look at the body as a machine, and sickness as a malfunction or failure of that machine. It works against the natural healing process by suppressing or masking symptoms. If trouble appears in one part, treatment is generally aimed at that part. The fact that physical disease is always integrated with emotion, life conditions, and other factors is generally not taken into account.

Fortunately, this perception of health is now beginning to change. But even if a medical doctor is ready to understand illness as a state of a whole, integrated organism, they have no options for treating it that way. Pharmaceutical drugs are developed to stop a particular expression of sickness, not to resolve its cause. Pharmaceutical protocols can only do what they are designed to do: force chemical changes in the body.

They are not, and *cannot be,* informed by a holistic view of human beings.

It can become necessary to take action against our own healing process when the natural healing force is overwhelmed, or when its reaction is excessive and endangers us. Conventional medicine has developed extraordinary interventions for emergency situations and severe illness. Contrary (or *allopathic*) treatment can be life-saving. But not everything is a life-or-death emergency. Acting against the vital energy, treating every health problem as an emergency—automatically, routinely, unnecessarily—is not without consequences.

All functions within a person are interrelated. Any type of intervention which forcefully manipulates the body's chemistry is best reserved for times when it is truly needed. There is universal consensus that a practitioner should "do no harm." The Hippocratic Oath affirms that when effective, safe, non-toxic options are available, they should be used first. Hippocrates, who is credited with first stating that rule, understood very well the interdependence of all aspects of a living being.

This fundamental difference in approach makes it clear why medical doctors view so many of today's complex chronic diseases as essentially hopeless. Faced with conditions which decimate quality of life, they often have no choice but to acknowledge that their arsenal of pharmaceuticals does not avail. In many cases, no matter how much they wish to give us good news and to help us be well, they can only repeat helplessly that the cause is unknown, and there is no cure.

It is critical that people begin to realize that such appraisals of illness do not represent objective fact, but an ideology: the belief system of one particular group of people. Most practitioners of conventional medicine are immersed in its peculiar doctrines. It is an intrinsically pessimistic methodology. In a world where healing and cure do happen every day, without drugs, theirs is not a reasonable outlook. We do not have the right to simply give up on natural healing when our unnatural interventions are harmful. No other type of healthcare, no other society, anywhere, at any time, has denied the central role of the inborn, always active tendency for rebalancing and healing.

Traditional medicines are more optimistic in general, because they embrace an incredibly powerful ally: life's continuous striving for health. They have been slowly, carefully built and refined over hundreds or thousands of years, always rooted in real-world observation, trial, and experience. Pharmaceuticals are always created in an environment very far removed from their application in a living human being. Their effects are studied in laboratories or in animals. Though much has been learned from them, animals are fundamentally different beings from humans, and both the logic and ethics of such studies are controversial.

Scientific study gives us ever more detailed information about the structure and functions of our bodies. The notion that the only way a person can recover from illness is by using synthetic drugs does not follow logically from that information. However, conventional medical knowledge, imaging, and other tests can provide a marvelously detailed picture of what is occuring in the physical body. Physiological clarity can help greatly, no matter what type of treatment we choose.

The ability to track changes over time, through blood work and other methods, can be of great benefit. For this reason, in many countries an integrated model of care has become more commonplace. For example, damage from chemotherapy can often be eased with nutritional and herbal protocols and homeopathic remedies. These natural therapies can also help with recovery after surgical or pharmaceutical interventions. Reducing side effects can help avoid additional medications.

Since billions of people have used, and continue to use, other types of healthcare with good results, we must open our minds and realize that conventional medicine is just one of many options available to us. Sometimes it's the best option; sometimes it has a collaborative part to play; sometimes it is unsuitable. Each type of healthcare has strengths and weaknesses. We are very fortunate to have several viable choices.

With the gift of choice comes the need for reliable information. Thinking through these ideas can help us decide which modality is most appropriate when we need help. This can be a particularly hard question when we have chronic health problems. Conventional care tends to focus on "managing sypmtoms." What does this really mean? It means trying to force the body to behave as if it is well, when it is letting us know very clearly that there's a problem—and perhaps a very deep problem. How could this be wise?

In classical homeopathy, a rational, coherent framework is in place for understanding what health is, and what the function of symptoms is. Its aim is not only recovery from the immediate symptoms, but the cultivation of better long-term health. It offers genuine hope, because it can increase the strength of the natural healing process. While the cause of a given condition may be a complete unknown in the view of a medical doctor, a homeopath can often see a different, more nuanced, and more comprehensive picture.

Consider the complexity and biological intelligence of a human being. Healing and regeneration happen so continuously in our bodies (and minds) that we take them for granted literally every moment of our lives. At least sixty times each minute your heart beats; every beat is a complex, finely orchestrated event which moves hundreds of billions of blood cells through your 60,000 miles of blood vessels. Nearly four million new cells come into being every second, as many are recycled to make room for them, and in less than a decade your entire body is remade. Yet you remain yourself, with your own unique memories, perceptions, identity. Each day you interact peacefully, often synergistically, with tens of thousands of different kinds of microbes. For all our curiosity, intellect, and technology, the processes governing life, and the forces that guide its development, are still very far beyond our understanding.

In truth, *all* medical systems are based on the fact that a living organism continually strives to correct imbalances and restore free, comfortable functioning. If this was not the case, medicine of any kind would be useless. Conventional medicine, homeopathy, and all the rest, depend on this reality. Once the chosen drug, or any other treatment, is administered, even the greatest team of doctors can only wait and hope that healing will occur.

We can make choices that facilitate healing, or that disrupt it; but the healing impulse will always be the work of nature. Homeopaths believe that rather than short-circuit the vital energy, we are wiser to respect it, learn from it, and assist it when necessary.

An intitial homeopathic consultation is long: typically ninety minutes to two hours. Follow-ups are often half an hour to an hour. Frequency of visits depends on the individual, but from four to eight weeks between appointments is common for someone with a chronic condition. In a calm and private environment, the homeopath gathers varied and detailed information.

In homeopathy, your whole lifetime is seen as an evolving health continuum. This is a crucial point of difference with conventional medicine, which tends to see problems which occur at different times, or in different organs, in isolation from the rest of the person's life—often even in isolation from the rest of their body.

A homeopath views the important events of life, including illness and medications, accidents, and emotional events, in terms of their lasting impact on health. If an illness is not truly cured, it can seem to disappear while it is actually developing into another condition. Careful attention is paid to your subjective understanding of your own experiences. The longer consultation and more relaxed pace are not simply a refreshing change but an important aspect of improving well-being. There is time for your questions; there is time for your unique situation to be explored in depth. Changes over time are considered carefully. The entire process encourages a growing self-reflection which gradually gives a new view of oneself and one's life.

Conventional medicine tends to keep patients in a comparatively passive state. Even the designation "patient" tells us something important about the roles that doctors and people who are sick usually play. More holistic systems can provide an opportunity (even the necessity) for a person who is ill to be much more active in the healing process. This in itself is strengthening. A homeopath often becomes a trusted mainstay of healthcare for several generations of a family.

That sort of relationship was the ideal of the family physician for centuries, but for the most part is now only a memory in conventional medicine. The impracticable "patient-load" and other demands are now too great. Of Canadian doctors interviewed in 2022, three quarters believed the quality of medical care patients were receiving had declined significantly in recent years. They were also dissatisfied with the fact that they spent almost two-thirds of their time on administrative tasks rather than working with patients.[6]

# 3
# Is a homeopath a naturopath or an herbalist?

A common misunderstanding is that homeopathy is the same as naturopathy or herbal medicine. In fact these are three distinct types of practice.

Naturopaths are graduates of specific naturopathic colleges. Their training includes some of the material of conventional medical school, but in addition they learn techniques of several traditional medical styles. They are knowledgable about nutrition and often treat health problems prioritizing diet, supplements, and herbs. These substances are generally much less toxic than pharmaceuticals, but still address symptoms primarily at the chemical level. Naturopathy may be seen as a compromise between conventional and natural medicines.

Naturopathic training also includes some study of both acupuncture and homopathy. However, these modalities are extremely complex and nuanced, and require years of specific study and mentored practice to become an expert practitioner.

Herbal medicine has countless variations. Using plants to relieve sufferings and encourage health is an age-old part of human life. There are many lineages and many different theoretical traditions. There is also great variation in the depth of understanding of herbal practitioners. The accessibility of the herbs themselves and information about their use is both a blessing and a potential problem. To practice herbalism with true experise requires lengthy study.

Like any other type of therapy, *how* herbs are used is important: herbs can be chosen to suppress symptoms. But as tonics and adaptogens herbs can be gently nutritive and can support healthy function and immunity. Nearly anyone can incorporate some health-protecting herbs into their daily life, and learn to use them to work through minor ailments. As always, a serious illness requires expert assessment and treatment. Gemmotherapy is a type of herbal medicine relatively unknown in North America, but wonderful to aquaint yourself with. It has a particular affinity for cleansing and regeneration of cells and tissues.

Many kinds of health care practitioners, including nutritional therapists, herbalists, naturopaths, osteopaths, and chiropractors wish to treat health problems at the deepest level possible. Many publicize their practice as doing so. But they don't always agree on what the source of sickness is. Where *is* the deepest level? Just as in conventional medicine, they often view disease as originating in a faulty organ, a dysfunction of an organ system, or a chemical imbalance.

To cite just a few examples: some believe that disease comes primarily from disturbance of the intestinal microbiome. Some believe nervous system dysfunction is the ultimate source of health problems; some say it's structural problems which must be corrected; some say it's hormone imbalance. Some cancers, for instance, are declared to be caused by estrogen dominance. Hay fever may be attributed to an intestinal impairment, or migraines to certain weather conditions or stress.

All of these ideas have merit and contain some truth. Various proposed cause-and-effect mechanisms may accurately describe a part of the disease process, once it has begun. But they do not explain how it began. Why did sickness appear in this form, in this person, at this moment in their life? They do not account for the fact that health and disease are extremely individual. Let's consider these conditions from a wider perspective.

Millions of people have similar stresses, but only a fraction—to use one of the examples mentioned above—develops a particular hormone imbalance. Of those who do, only a fraction will then develop a certain form of cancer. So while there is value in the insight, it is describing a fairly advanced stage in the disease process. The hormone imbalance is not a fundamental cause but a symptom produced along the way. If we aim treatment at the hormonal system, we have not addressed the cause of the disease and will not heal the susceptibility or deeper distress.

The perspective of classical homeopathy is that all of these disturbances in the body are manifestations of a deeper, energetic disturbance. Their specific forms depend upon the individual. The remedies reach very deeply into an organism; but the conditions in which we live certainly influence our immunity. The more we can remove obstacles to healing, the more successful homeopathic treatment is likely to be.

To look at another of our examples, most people in industrialized nations have compromised intestinal health, yet of the millions who breathe in pollen each day, only a small minority overreact with the symptoms of hay fever. If changes in barometric pressure or stress (or any of the other common triggers) were the *cause* of migraines, all of us would suffer migraines. Homeopathy correctly applied may be able to resolve the person's vulnerability to the trigger. Their tendency to experience an exaggerated reaction to normal conditions can be reduced or, often, completely resolved.

The expressions of illness are tremendously varied. They include not only physical sickness but emotional, cognitive, and social manifestations. And there are people who remain robustly healthy even in extremely poor circumstances. Clearly there is something highly individual at work in health and sickness.

These other therapies differ from homeopathy in that they are mostly constrained within the biochemical model of disease. Many traditions understand that the physical, mental, and emotional aspects of a person are an integrated whole, but their interventions are still chemical or mechanical. Herbs and foods do have an energetic effect, as does the relief of misalignment or excessive tension in the body. These treatments can indeed be helpful in some cases, but may not be specifically attuned enough to the individual, at a deep enough level, for permanent, decisive healing.

Of the healthcare systems commonly available to us today, expertly applied acupuncture and homeopathy may be the deepest-acting therapies. Acupuncture can have a direct effect on a relevant part of the energy system; a correctly chosen homeopathic remedy has a uniquely individualized precision. From the point of view of a homeopath, the susceptibility to both good health and illness, and even our identity, emerge from a deeper level than chemistry. We are all made of the same substances, organized in exactly the same ways. Why, then, are we all unique? As an energy medicine, homeopathy recognizes that energetic fields underlie everything about us, giving us our characteristic traits and tendencies, from our DNA to our fears to our favorite foods. The scientific confirmation of this will be discussed in a later chapter.

An energetic disturbance can manifest itself in the physical, emotional, psychological, or cognitive life of a person—or any combination of those. Such a disturbance can persist for many years, or even for the whole lifetime. A human life begins before birth, literally submerged in the chemistry of another person and with the inheritance of many generations. An energetic injury or disorder may begin in utero. In fact, most probably, all modern people are born with some disturbance in the energetic level (we will see more about this in the next chapter). Treating a disease at the physical or mental level, in other words at the level of the manifestation, is at best *rearranging* the disease. Restoring order at the energetic level allows a natural, spontaneous emergence of true health.

# 4

# Why would I try homeopathic healthcare?

Many factors prompt people to try homeopathy. Most often, they have already tried both conventional medicine and other alternatives. Typically they have experienced disappointment or frustration after using conventional medicine for years without real improvement, in some cases finding themselves worse off than before treatment. As was touched on earlier, conventional medicine is not equipped, in its ideology or its treatment options, to generate systemic health. That simply is not what it is designed to do.

Those who wish to pursue healing at a deep level must sooner or later look for alternatives, so it is no surprise that there is an accelerating migration at this time toward natural healthcare. Homeopathy is a particularly gentle and unobtrusive option with transformative power in many cases. This chapter will explore some positive impacts of homeopathic medicine. It will also open some larger topics which are uncomfortable for many of us. There is a message we need to be open to: the feedback we're receiving from our bodies, our societies, and our environment, is that our choices in healthcare have a much wider sphere of influence than just our own comfort and well-being.

A very common reason people look to homeopathy is the toxicity of pharmaceuticals. The harms caused by drugs are referred to as "side" effects, as if they are trivial inconveniences, rather than real symptoms of a new, iatrogenic syndrome. And although each drug is accompanied by a long list of possible complications, those lists include only the ones which are obvious and appear quickly. There is no information about what the more subtle or long-term effects might be. Everyone is an individual, with unique predispositions and sensitivities, and will be affected in different ways.

Referring to these new symptoms as side effects induces the patient to accept them as an inevitable part of trying to get well. When people begin to question that very questionable assumption, they usually start investigating alternative medicines. While this might be a good idea, remember that if you are using prescription medication and would like to change to another kind of healthcare, it's critical that you talk with your doctor about it. Do not stop your medications without medical guidance. If you consult with an alternative practitioner (who is not also a doctor) who tells you to do so, they are overstepping what safety and the law allow.

Pharmaceutical drug use, which dominates conventional care, presents many other pressing concerns as well. All of them are becoming more urgent with each passing year: contaminated medications; antibiotic and antiviral resistance; overdose; addiction; misdiagnosis; dispensing errors; tremendous ecological harm; and the list could continue. Putting all of these together, the people who suffer adverse effects each year in North America number in the millions (including hundreds of thousands of deaths). Pondering all of this reveals the urgent need to think hard about our current trajectory. These issues impact not just each of us individually, but whole societies, and the world beyond human societies.

One of the difficulties is that pharmaceuticals are inherently unsafe. Another is the evident overwhelm of the medical system. The present model is not working well for staff or for patients. Some seem to believe we are trapped in this downward spiral, as if nothing can be done differently and no other options exist. This is an untruth from which more and more people are freeing themselves. Everyone would benefit if the conventional system was relieved of cases which could be resolved through alternative means. This would leave medical resources for those who truly need them. The quality of care they receive would undoubtedly rise, as would the health and morale of doctors, nurses, and other staff.

From a holistic point of view, there is another serious concern. When a disturbance is suppressed, rather than actually resolved, it will emerge again in another form. With repeated suppressions, the forms it takes become increasingly severe. Suppression through medication means chemically forcing the body (or mind) to stop manifesting evidence of its distress. We know quite well in other contexts that suppressing a problem only intensifies the harm—think of emotional trauma, or social injustice. The same is true in our health. This seems to be a matter of natural law.

The question of *when* illness is recognized is key. We all realize that we have a better chance of healing if we begin our efforts earlier in the disease process. In this, conventional medicine is limited: because it only recognizes isolated symptoms which fit into standardized diagnoses, by the time a doctor can identify a disease it has been developing for years and is much harder to treat successfully. Screening for disease is of course intended to be preventative. But the reality is that by the time those tests find pathological change, such as a tumor or tissues destroyed by autoimmune activity, the disturbance has been evolving for a long time and may have powerful momentum. But there are ways to see problems developing in earlier stages, often before the immune system is so weakened that it becomes unable prevent that destructive momentum.

Where a medical doctor may see a number of unrelated, meaningless symptoms over a period of years or even decades, a classical homeopath recognizes a progression. We can progress into disease: from relatively superficial problems to more severe, hard to treat, even life-threatening pathologies. But in many cases, with care oriented toward restoring and sustaining natural healing capacities, we can progress from disease into the richness and relief of good health.

Research shows (and common sense agrees) that dietary, chemical, environmental, and emotional stresses alter our genetic expression in ways that directly influence our health. We know as well that these alterations may be inherited by the generations which follow us. The branch of biology called *epigenetics* studies this in depth. Researchers have recently begun to examine the epigenetic harm that medications are causing.[7] Their findings offer some explanation for the fact that human immune systems are now weaker with each new generation.

When pharmaceuticals became the predominant form of medical treatment in the twentieth century, there was a period of diminishing mortality rates from infectious disease. Of course this brought tremendous relief and was rightly celebrated. But it should give us pause to consider that since that time there has been an extraordinarily steep increase in degenerative, inflammatory, immune-related diseases.

Suffering from mental and emotional health problems and rates of infertility have also increased drastically. A host of disorders which were rare or even unknown have become commonplace. Every generation is more severely afflicted than the one before, and sickness steadily claims people at younger ages.

Homeopathic care is one of the choices people make to reverse these frightening trends, to move toward restoring immunity and quality of life. Successful natural medicine alters our genetic expression for the better, and these changes too are heritable. The "defeat" of infectious disease by antibiotics has been one of the most promoted accomplishments of conventional medicine, but that achievement is now being reversed due to the surge of antibiotic-resistant pathogens. Homeopathy has treated infectious disease successfully for over two hundred years, including cholera, typhoid, diptheria, influenza, SARS viruses, and many others.

Homeopathic remedies are non-toxic in the human body and in the environment. This stands in contrast to conventional medications: the manufacture, use, and disposal of drugs have created a surge of ecological damage. More than 100,000 metric tons of drugs are used each year, which then are released into the biosphere.[8] Infectious materials, hormones, radioactive and other hazardous products have found their way into water supplies and living bodies in every corner of the world. During the early years of the Covid-19 pandemic, an estimated 16,650 tons of additional biomedical pollution accumulated every day.[9]

Economic sustainability is also a pressing concern. The average cost to develop a new drug (known as an "asset,") is around 2.23 billion US dollars,[10] and up to $4.46 billion.[11] Many quickly become obsolete or are withdrawn. In 2021, 18 million Americans could not afford the medications they had been prescribed, and in Canada, while some medical costs are covered by provincial plans, drug costs are not, creating a terrible economic strain on sick people and their families. Often the cost of medications is simply prohibitive. Untreated disease leads to myriad negative consequences.

Most of the important homeopathic remedies have remained unchanged for two hundred years. They will never need to be updated or reformulated. Their safety is proven beyond any shadow of doubt. They are made from free whole natural substances, in minute quantities. A commonly used remedy such as Sulphur (made from the pure mineral) or Staphysagria (made from a common flowering plant) will never be the property of any individual or company. Alhough in most circumstances it would be laborious and impractical, it is technically possible for anyone to make these remedies with a tiny pinch of the raw material and a few basic tools. Profit has never been a factor in the their development; there is no formula to hide or patent.

There is now, unfortunately, an exception to this: the recent flood of combination remedies which have become available to the public. Their marketing is targeted for people who like the idea of a natural solution but are not well informed about how homeopathy works. These combination products sell well, because they seem to provide the quick fix modern people often expect. But there are important problems associated with taking combination remedies. This question will be examined closely in Chapter Eleven.

A healthcare approach which strengthens your constitution and immunity, a treatment which leaves you in improved physical, emotional, and cognitive health, means less need for medical treatment in the future. The United States has spent more than $4.5 trillion on healthcare in recent years and insurance companies are seeing their profits (which they measure in trillions of dollars) rise in double digits. Yet we steadily have more disease, not less.

Imagine, please, the myriad benefits if even a small fraction of the resources that are poured into the mainstream healthcare system and drug development went to providing access to natural alternatives. Imagine the personal and the population-wide health benefits of avoiding unneccessary toxicity, for the present and for the future.

Emotional and psychological illness are epidemic. The strains and imbalances of modern life are taking a heavy toll. Our consciousness now carries constant awareness of problems that are global in scale. Generations of suppressed physical disease have relentlessly forced disturbances deeper, creating more complex physical pathologies and increased pressure and suffering in the mental and emotional spheres.

Use of mental health services and psychotherapy have risen hugely. In part this is probably because it's now more socially acceptable to take care of your psychological health. But the number and magnitude of stressors has certainly increased as well. Antidepressant use has risen steeply, especially in children and younger adults.

Public awareness of the importance of mental health has exploded—it is discussed everywhere you look. America's mental health crisis cost $282 billion in 2024 alone.[12] And yet, as noted with physical sickness, more treatment has not created more health. Rather, in the same time frame the problem has increased. Rates of suicide have risen drastically, as much as thirty percent since 2000.[13]

The predominant strategy in conventional medicine of trying to silence pain and disorder threatens our very existence. Living organisms simply do not *heal* from the outside in. Drugs often put further pressure on an already overstressed system. Homeopathy has always recognized that mental and emotional health are of the greatest importance. Our capacity for happiness, good relationships, humor, meaningful work, even our identity can be decimated by emotional and psychological pain. The aim of a classical homeopath is always to regenerate health from the deepest levels.

In complicated or severe cases, a combination of therapies may be needed. Changing, reducing, or stopping a medication must be done with great care and under the supervision of an appropriate medical provider. Sometimes stopping is neither safe nor appropriate. But as people, and as a society, we need to understand that a pharmaceutical drug cannot bring true healing to these illnesses. This is a known fact: doctors don't talk in term of curing severe mental illness, but in terms of managing it. Does that mean there's no hope? No; it means we need to become wiser about human health and about medicine.

Talk therapies can undoubtedly help in some cases, but talk usually does not reach the depth at which the disturbance is active. Analyzing or describing one's emotional pain may be important sometimes, to learn about the origin and expression of the problem, or for relief from the pressure and pain. Often after a psychotherapy session, a person feels improvement, but back in ordinary life, their distress overtakes them again. This might continue for many years. The relief is real, and of course that is a good thing! Yet it often does not truly resolve the trouble.

To look at it in another light, describing the sensation of pain from a broken limb doesn't heal the bone. Taking a painkiller is completely reasonable but also does not mend the fracture. Thinking and talking about trauma or mental illness will not always bring healing to deep psychological conditions. We assume that healing an emotional wound must take years of therapy and be very difficult. But that is not always true; we assume so because most of us have never had a treatment which relieved the trauma directly.

Therapies such as Emotional Freedom Techniques (EFT) can often bring deep resolution stunningly quickly. Why? EFT meets the trauma or anxiety where it lives, so to speak: in the underlying energetic system. When combined with energy medicine in this way, psychotherapy can actually become much more useful. EFT is so effective because it works with the energy meridians established by traditional Asian medicines. For the same reason, energy therapies like acupuncture and homeopathy can greatly increase the benefit of the work you do with a psychotherapist.

In the case stories related at the end of this book, you will see examples of healing in the *direction of cure*. When healing and strengthening happen first at the deepest level, the disturbance can gradually move to less vital parts. As the whole organism gains strength, good health can be manifested from the inside out.

# 5
# What is the origin of homeopathy?

In the early nineteenth century, homeopathy's founders were medical doctors who had lost faith in the accepted protocols of their day: harsh and dangerous treatments such as excessive bloodletting, deliberately burning the skin to create blisters, and prescriptions of harsh purgatives and known poisons like arsenic, lead, and mercury which caused permanent damage or, quite frequently, death.

Samuel Hahnemann was a German doctor, chemist, and scholar. When he witnessed the lasting harm from these treatments, he closed his medical practice in a crisis of conscience. But he was irresistibly drawn back into medicine. While translating ancient texts (he was proficient in at least nine languages) he came across clues for a wholly different approach: similar medicine. He began methodically conducting experiments on himself with tiny, stimulating doses of herbs, researching the principle of similarity. He carefully recorded every detail of the process. Gradually using more and more dilute doses, his results were so encouraging that he soon attracted a working group of like-minded physicians and other professionals. The real breakthrough came when he found that a certain way of processing the medicinal solution, what he termed *potentizing*, somehow greatly magnified its healing potential while completely eliminating toxicity (potentizing will be explained in a later chapter).

This team advanced homeopathy by painstaking, thorough investigation and documentation of one mineral or plant extract at a time. The early homeopaths were the first Western physicians to insist there must be a rational, consistent theory of health and disease, upon which a reliable basis for medical practice could be built. Searching for ways to make the "new medicine" as dependable and well-grounded as possible, they invented the placebo-controlled study. It became (and remains, for classical homeopaths) the backbone of new remedy discovery and development.

As waves of epidemic disease devastated Europe, homeopathy was many times more successful in curing and preventing infection than the haphazard, often superstitious treatments of the time.[14] Government and hospital records show the dramatic differences. For example, while conventional doctors were losing more than half their patients in the cholera epidemic of the 1830s, homeopathic doctors lost as few as five percent in the same cities.[15,]

The success in treatment (and in some instances prevention) of epidemic disease helps to explain the rapid early conversion of many doctors to homeopathy. This is a pattern we still see today: many homeopaths begin as medical doctors who undertake additional training when experience shows them the benefits of homeopathic care.

Hahnemann was a controversial figure in his own time. He was outspoken, adamant about the need to evolve medicine and provide safer, more humane treatments. He wrote publicly to his colleagues, proclaiming that diet was an important factor in health and immunity, and he insisted on hygienic practices to prevent the spread of infectious diseases.[16] Both of these were radical ideas at the time and his recommendations were met with outrage and ridicule.

Hahnemann also insisted that people suffering from mental and emotional illness or trauma must be treated with the same compassion and respect as those with physical disease.[17] This was a direct challenge to the medical establishment (and society in general) which saw persons with mental and emotional symptoms as sinners, criminals, souls possessed by the devil, or at best as hopelessly impaired. Hahnemann achieved some famous cures in such cases which brought yet more doctors asking to be taught his new medicine.

Over the following decades, homeopaths' labors helped to change perceptions of mental illness. When homeopathy reached the United States, comfortable, compassionate recovery centers for the mentally ill were established. There followed an era of great progress in these facilities, led by innovative homeopaths working together with open-minded medical staff.[18] They were shut down in the early twentieth century when it became unacceptable, even criminal, to treat any kind of illness through means other than chemical drugs or surgery. This was deeply unfortunate as the field of mental health was set back grievously. It has yet to fully recover from that reversal.

The nineteenth century was an era of extraordinary advancement in the sciences, and Hahnemann was a consummate scientist. His thinking was unusually broad, encompassing multiple disciplines. He developed a sophisticated theory of heretitary predisposition after many years of observing patterns of infection and the characteristic impacts they caused in subsequent generations. This was long before any coherent theory of genetics existed. Even the concept of the gene was still to come.

The Augustinian clergyman Gregor Mendel, highly educated in mathematics and science, systematically experimented with breeding garden peas for different flower color, seed shape, and other traits. His work is considered the first scientific study of heritable traits. He could only attribute what he saw to "invisible factors." But he had opened the way for the new science of genetics. He published his results in 1865. The following year Ernst Haeckel coined the term "ecology" to describe another new field of study: the influence of environment on human evolution (our use of the word has changed somewhat since then).

Hahnemann published his theories on hereditary predisposition in 1828, almost four decades before Mendel and Haeckel formulated their ideas. In his book, *The Chronic Diseases,* he explored the multigenerational impacts of environment, disease, and trauma on human health. Although the language of his books may feel outmoded today, Hahnemann's works are infused with surprisingly relevant, modern notions of social justice, sustainability, and ethics. Each of us has a purpose, he believed, to improve ourselves and contribute as much as we can, however we can, "for the common good." The better our health, the more compassionate we will be, and the wiser our decisions will be.

Within a single generation, homeopathy spread throughout Europe and beyond. By the early 1900s it had enjoyed a century of popularity in North America, where there were dozens of homeopathic hospitals and colleges. Gradually they closed under pressure from the American Medical Association and changes in goverment policy, lobbied for by tycoons with vested interests in the fast-expanding chemical drug industry. The transformation was underway to the medical industrial complex we see today. Only an officially sanctioned, narrowly defined biochemical model was to be permitted in healthcare.

With the loss of its schools, homeopathic medicine nearly disappeared from North America. But about half a century later a revival of classical homeopathy began in Europe, fueled largely by the renewal of Hahnemann's work by a few dedicated individuals. In the twenty-first century it is growing again in North America, far past what those early converts to the new medicine could have imagined.

# 6
# How does it work?

To understand what a homeopathic remedy does, we have to consider what a living organism is doing, both in a state of health and in sickness. As an example, imagine you have caught a flu and you have a fever and a cough. Before you got sick, you didn't have symptoms. Your immune system was in a more relaxed state; it wasn't actively trying to defend against a virus.

Now you feel ill, but the virus is not causing your symptoms. The symptoms are mechanisms your body uses to help eliminate the virus. The virus isn't causing your fever; the vital energy has raised your body temperature because this inhibits the growth of the virus. The virus isn't causing your cough either. Coughing is a way of expelling the pathogen, as are sneezing or a running nose. Body aches and sore throat are sensations of inflammation. These days inflammation is usually spoken of as a problem, and chronic inflammation is a problem—one of our greatest population-wide health problems. However, the inflammatory process serves a vitally important purpose in acute conditions, like an infection or an injury. This is common knowledge in conventional medicine, and yet the automatic reaction is to suppress it. No consideration is given to what that suppression means to the organism.

Symptoms, uncomfortable as they can be, are intelligent responses to a stress of some kind. We have been culturally primed to fear them, but they are there to protect us from worse consequences—in this example, from worsening infection. The particular qualities of your symptoms show what strategies your defense mechanism is using to bring you back to health. Just as we have individual personalities, we react in different ways to life's challenges, including sickness.

Some of your friends may be infected with the same virus, but their symptoms will not be identical to yours. One person might be feeling chilly, weak, trembling, and complain of a terrible headache, yet they feel slightly better if they sit outside in the fresh air. Another might be flushed, extremely thirsty, aching, and sluggish. A third might feel chilled, suffering with nausea, wanting reassuring company and conversation, and drinking lots of cold water. If you go to a doctor with your flu, it will almost certainly not occur to them to consider your mood, what you are craving to eat while you're sick, or how a change of temperature makes you feel. But these are expressions of an organism which can help in the choice of a homeopathic remedy. After all, you, a whole person, are coping with the flu, not just some of your cells. It's you, that whole you, the remedy is for. A homeopath will recognize a different remedy indicated for you and each of your friends.

Respecting the innate healing tendency, and also the individuality of the person who is ill, a classical homeopath will choose a remedy which gives the vital force extra energy to achieve its purpose. This is why when you take the correct remedy for your flu, you will probably first experience a slight increase of one or more symptoms, after which your recovery can surprisingly rapid and complete. In the process, your immune system is strengthened.

A useful analogy to envision why this works is the resonance of sound waves. A vibration of a certain frequency produces a particular pitch. When a musician tunes her instrument to a tuning fork, she can hear dissonance when it is out of tune. As she adjusts the instrument, she is gradually altering the frequency until it becomes perfectly resonant with that emitted by the tuning fork. When they suddenly match, the change is unmistakable. This is very much like the experience of taking a correct homeopathic remedy. When the work of the vital force is amplified this way, energy can flow more freely, facilitating healing.

For the same flu, you and your friends would all be given the same conventional medications (including over-the-counter drugs) aimed at halting your symptoms by interfering with the efforts of your immune system. They would force your body temperature down, prevent the removal of the pathogen through coughing. Their job is to override and suppress the protective, healing response. This prolongs the sickness, and it confuses and weakens the immune system. It creates a state of inner dissonance. In such a medium, it's harder for the subtle communication networks of your body to work with clarity. It's harder for energy to flow.

The stronger your immune system is, the more it may resist the suppression and produce symptoms. You then take more of the medication, or different one, to fight against the new expression of the organism. If you do this often enough, or if you happen to be sensitive to those drugs, your immune system will be damaged, whether suddenly or gradually. For someone whose constitution is already weakened, it can preciptate disaster. Even in a strong organism, it degrades the ability to maintain health. This may show up in more frequent and longer infections; or it may harm your immune system so much that it can't even react or create symptoms anymore. When I hear someone say "I never get sick," I see it as a matter for concern.

Healing systems throughout the world and thoughout human history have affirmed that all organisms live, grow, heal, and bring offspring into the world—every single one unique—due to the presence of a vital, animating force or energy. Until very recently science, religion or spirituality, and medicine were not seen as separate. In much of the world, this is still the case. Even in countries with a strong emphasis on modern healthcare, their connection is evident, a matter of common sense, to many people.

A few hundred years ago, a strange new idea began to gain traction in the West: the notion that the natural world and all living things operate purely mechanically. In this view there is no vital force, nor does life have direction or purpose; we humans and all other living beings are, quite literally, machines. (Obviously this raises big questions, such as: how did all this machinery get here, and what impetus keeps it going? And many others which are beyond the scope of this book.)

There is a curious legend about the way this belief came to dominate our culture, and to define our version of science. René Descartes is said to have bargained with the Roman Catholic Church: he would be permitted to study the human body, to catalogue its anatomy, if he did not trouble the soul, which belonged to God. The separation of body from soul allowed the study of living bodies to begin in earnest—with the dead. Among other precedents set when science and religion parted ways, it became established that the way to learn about how living things work is to examine isolated parts of them, when they are no longer living and working. In counterpoint to this, the way of traditional medicines has generally been to cultivate great sensitivity to the living and working.

Though it may sound like a simplistic fable to modern ears, the fiction of a total division between body and soul, a pact of sorts between the Church and investigators of nature (whether it was a formal agreement or not) took root. In the small world of a new discipline, which would come to be called *science*, the idea became deeply embedded. Such things as spirit, soul, or even a life force or vital energy, if they existed at all, were not to contaminate science. Whatever it is that gives life had nothing to do with even biology, which literally translates to "study of life!" Ultimately, it was taken so absurdly far as to deny the existence of a living energy in living beings.

The modern disciplines of biology and biochemistry were build on this dubious foundation, and today many scientists never think to question it. Their textbooks presented concepts only within established boundaries. If they do deviate from the paradigm, they risk censure from their peers, loss of funding, and can even find themselves unemployed and unemployable. But there are always some who have the common sense and courage to question artificial restrictions on thought. There is no reason why the dynamics of life can't be included in scientific study. And there is now, at last, strong movement in that direction.

However, education in the mainstream life sciences perpetuates old ideas. The dogmatic still reject the idea of a vital force sustaining life and health, because we can't see, weigh, and measure it. Yet they offer no alternative explanation. The reality of an adaptive, healing activity is obvious and easily observed in every living thing, from a bacterium to an elephant to an oak tree. And when life leaves a body, no one can be in any doubt that a profound, irreversible change has taken place. All of the chemical constituents remain, but the vital energy no longer animates them. Something has left the body; very quickly its order disintegrates.

It has been well demonstrated by scientific research that the human body generates complex, highly ordered energy fields and channels. This is not pseudoscience; these profound discoveries have given rise to a new branch of science: biofield physiology.[19] In this domain, scientists are beginning to understand healing systems such as acupuncture and homeopathy. There should be nothing surprising in the fact that disturbance of these energy fields (which we *can* see and measure)[20,21] provokes discomfort and dysfunction. It follows that healing therapies would, ideally, work at that energetic level.

"Symptoms" are efforts to restore order and energy flow. The vital force keeps the disturbance as far as possible from the most vital parts of the organism. Homeopathy helps it overcome, adapt, evolve into a new state of order. Even the conventional medical model takes for granted that the body is maintained by a self-organizing force which constantly maintains homeostasis and extraordinarily complex functions, to which the changes it considers mistakes or failures of the body, experienced as illness or pain, are exceptions.

A strange, irrational resistance is perpetuated in conventional medicine to acknowledging that its interventions are also ultimately reliant on a natural healing process which is not within our direct control. No doubt this is due in part to the wide gap between pure research and the everyday affairs of medical schools, pharmacies, government agencies, insurance companies, and doctors' offices. It always takes a long time for advances in knowledge to trickle down, especially since medical school research and curriculum, as well as continuing education and personal guidance for physicians, are sponsored or otherwise influenced, in a perennial ethical no-man's-land, by pharmaceutical companies.[22,23,24] And it is no doubt quite hard for many deeply committed doctors (among others) to embrace the fact that we will never be fully in control of sickness and health. Belief that we can establish such control may be benevolent delusion, but it is delusion nonetheless.

Many traditional medical practitioners, homeopaths, martial artists, people well practiced in meditation or religious contemplation, and others have intimate familiarity with the human organism as an energetic system as well as a chemical system. It's quite clear from scientific study, millennia of experimentation and experience, and plain common sense, that a person comprises both. Only when the energy flow is well ordered and unobstructed can good health on the chemical level follow.

We know that every experience, and every substance, encountered will cause effects throughout an organism (or ecosystem), to a greater or lesser extent. Strong experiences and substances can cause important and lasting effects, even permanent changes, including death—or cure. This fact offers more precise insight into the prevalence of immune disorders and degenerative diseases in modern, developed societies. It's no coincidence that their populations are the most out of touch with natural living and natural healing.

Weathly countries with the most advanced medical technology, and the easiest access to it, consistently have the highest rates of complicated, perplexing chronic degenerative diseases. For many generations now our well-being and our ability to cope with challenges has been eroded by a barrage of stresses: toxins in air, water, and food; powerful synthetic medications; radically unnatural diets; even loss of connection to the natural rhythms of light and darkness. There is no one reason for all of the health problems we face today, nor is there one simple solution. But surely it makes sense to minimize exposure to these stresses when we can, especially when better alternatives are readily available.

Classical homeopathy is based on a few simple, timeless principles or natural laws. One of these is known as the *law of similars.* For thousands of years medical scholars around the world have noted that when a large dose of a substance causes symptoms of illness, a minute dose of it stimulates healing of the same symptoms. This concept was known to Hahnemann from his study of medical history and ancient texts. Hundreds, if not thousands, of examples of similar prescribing are found across virtually all types of medicine.

In fact, there are many conventional drugs which work on this principle as well, though it is rarely explicitly recognized. Doctors generally are unaware when their prescriptions fall under this law; some drugs are descended from older medical and herbal traditions. But modern science knows well that it is a common property of biological systems (part of a realm of biology called hormesis)[25]. A large quantity poisons; a tiny quantity stimulates healing.

As an example, we can consider digitalis, a common flowering plant (also known as foxglove). It has been used for thousands of years as a medicinal herb. It can be problematic in herbal medicine and must be used with care, since the plant is toxic. For almost a century there has been a pharmaceutical drug derived from the plant, which is used primarily for cardiac problems.

In accordance with the law of similars, the side effects of this drug correspond to the poisoning symptoms of the plant: shortness of breath, edema, nausea and gastrointestinal problems, cardiac symptoms, unusual visual disturbances, general weakness, mental confusion, and a great many others. Classical homeopaths also use a remedy made from digitals, in a high-dilution, potenized form—a stimulating, energetic dose—to heal those symptoms, which were revealed in its homeopathic *proving*. The remedy is free of side effects.

Hahnemann devised a way to study the energetic effects of a substance. If he could see the syndrome (the characteristic set of symptoms) which it provoked, he reasoned, that would tell him what symptoms it had the potential to cure. The study model he created is known as a proving. It involves observing the reactions of healthy people to the potentized substance. The experiment is to be conducted in stable, healthy volunteers.

The proving process begins long before anyone takes the remedy, however, with weeks of careful documentation of the sensations, moods, sleep and thought patterns, even food preferences and aversions that are normal for each prover. This step is essential because it allows any new symptoms to be clearly discerned. The provers take just enough of the remedy to stimulate changes. Neither the provers nor the supervisors who collect data from them daily know what substance is being proved. The provers' reactions—of every sort—are recorded over a period of months or even years.

In addition to the results of provings, any reliable historical observations of the substance are taken into account, such as hospital records. A common poisonous plant or a toxic material which people have been exposed to in building, mining, or industry often has a long history of accidental poisonings. The most consistent symptoms they have produced help to confirm the remedy's characteristics. Over time a rich, multi-faceted "picture" of the substance appears. Analysis of clinical case studies further expands the knowledge. There is a never-ending effort to increase the understanding.

When you consult a classical homeopath, they will gather a lot of information about you, not only symptoms of sickness. They are attempting to see the whole dynamic expression the vital force is making as it works to restore your health. That totality will be matched with the remedy which contains the most similar expressions. In this way the law of similars underpins homeopathic practice.

Another core principle of homeopathy is the use of only one remedy at a time. This is why classical homeopaths are also called *unicist* (or sometimes *Hahnemannian*) homeopaths. The totality, or the coherent picture of the vital energy expressing itself through you, can again be imagined as a particular frequency. The remedy also represents a whole, unique, coherent frequency. The aim is the greatest possible agreement between the two. They will not be exactly the same—it's *similar* medicine, not *identical*—but the closer they are, the more the remedy can amplify the action of the vital energy, and the quicker and more complete will be the healing.

In time—maybe a short time, maybe much longer—the person's whole picture is likely to change. This new image then needs to be considered carefully, and the next remedy chosen. A few people may have such a strong affinity for a certain remedy that no matter what kind of illness they have, it will indicate that same remedy. This is known as a person's *constitutional* remedy. There is fairly strong consensus among most homeopaths that the phenomenon of a person needing only one constitutional remedy all their lives is much less common now than it was in Hahnemann's time. This is due to the increased exposure over the generations to unnatural lifestyles and diets, powerful environmental toxins and suppressive medications, and other factors. The epigenetic changes from these pressures has complicated immunity and made it harder for the vital force to produce a clear, consistent signal.

The third fundamental principle of homeopathy is that remedy is individualized. The *similimum,* the most similar remedy, can be found only by matching the unique state of *this* person, at *this* time.

A number of people may have the same medical diagnosis; a medical doctor will have a limited set of protocols to choose from for each diagnosis. But a homeopath has many hundreds of remedies available which should be considered. Even if the people have all have received the same diagnosis, their whole state will not be the same.

As well, one might need frequent repetition of a low potency of a remedy, while another might need just one dose in a higher potency. One may then need a different remedy, or a repetition of the same remedy, or a rest from remedies.

The fourth rule is the use of the smallest dose which is effective. A remedy is intended to be stimulating, not forceful. This is most efficiently accomplished by using the *minimum dose.* Once the energy system has received the stimulus of the remedy, it must be allowed to do its work. In classical homeopathy, the aim is never to pressure or short-circuit the natural healing process or to try to outsmart the organism.

The principle of the minimum dose is a simple idea, but some mental adjustment is needed when one is used to conventional medical prescriptions which are meant to be taken continuously for weeks, months, or even a lifetime. The first homeopaths were highly aware of the potential negative effects of medications; it was a primary motivation for their work. For many years, Hahnemann and his team patiently tested smaller and smaller doses, intent on developing the safest possible medicine.

One of Hahnemann's great leaps of insight was a method of processing the remedies which increased the effectiveness while minimizing the dose. Potentizing, his revolutionary discovery, will be discussed in the next chapter. It seems counterintuitive that the more dilute a remedy is, the more powerfully and deeply it acts within a human organism. But this is what was found with great consistency.

Hahnemann had stumbled upon phenomena which are only now beginning to be understood. Science itself has grown so much that we now know reality is full to overflowing with the counterintuitive: quantum physics shows us that fundamental aspects of nature do indeed feel impossibly bewildering when we first encounter them.

# 7
# Is there scientific research on homeopathy?

The answer to this question is a resounding *yes*. Today, ongoing work in all the major sciences is bringing a whole new dimension to the accepted view of health and disease. Biology, chemistry, pharmacology, even physics, have drawn closer together as each advances individually. All of them are now providing pieces of the homeopathic puzzle.

This is a difficult time for humanity: many conditions which were rare (or non-existent) have become very common. Millions of people live with debilitating pain and limitation. Anxiety and depression accompany the violence and destruction we hear about, or experience directly, each day. Yet we are poised in a tremendously optimistic moment for healthcare, if we open our minds to a more holistic understanding of what health is, and what we want medicine to be. Yes: it's up to us.

Recent scientific studies have led to more widespread acceptance of many traditional medicines and practices. Of course, their efficacy never depended upon whether mainstream scientists accepted them or not. But for many who are uncertain what kind of healthcare they want, new understanding of how and why they work may give more confidence to try different alternatives. In pursuing their own research trajectories, scientific disciplines which dismissed traditional medicines are now independently discovering the principles which have always underlain acupuncture, homeopathy, and other therapies. The concepts of energy medicine are becoming mainstream.

There is a very large, rapidly growing body of research on homeopathy, from around the world. There are two distinct streams of research. Fundamental research is exploring the materials and the mechanisms of action of the remedies. Clinical research is studying the outcomes of homeopathy in practice.

Hundreds of clinical studies support classical homeopathy as a safe, effective method of healthcare. There are organizations working to make them available and approachable for the general public, including Americans for Homeopathy Choice, Homeopathy Research Institute, and Research In Homeopathy.[26,27,28]

Because it approaches sickness so differently from conventional medicine, homeopathy requires appropriate studies to be realistically evaluated. Conventional drugs are intended to lessen or eliminate particular symptoms, so they are tested in relation to the reduction of those symptoms. For homeopathic remedies to give satisfactory results, they are *not* prescribed by those criteria. Nor can their success or failure be measured in the same ways. Therefore studies which simply swap one kind of prescription for the other are meaningless and misleading. As one homeopath put it, you don't expect to measure an object's weight with a ruler.

The true, realistic results appear when the remedies are studied as they are intended to be used in practice: selected for each individual and their unique situation. The subjective experience of the person who is sick is routinely ignored in clinical medical studies as irrelevant; chemical changes in a particular tissue are the holy grail. But in homeopathy a person's experience of their own well-being is an important marker.

The beneficial results of homeopathic medicine have been known since the beginning, but until recently we didn't have technologies which could approach the fundamental research. We had no way to actually see and measure the material and action of the remedies.

There were various hypotheses about the contents of extreme dilutions, but they could not be tested in a laboratory (though they were meticulously tested in human beings). With the astoundingly sensitive tools available today, this has changed. A surge of energy is going into homeopathy research in many countries, making use of these advanced technologies. But science and homeopathy are not new to each other.

Samuel Hahnemann saw that something was occuring, in an absolutely consistent way, in life on Earth. All living organisms would heal spontaneously if they had sufficient energy and favorable conditions. Yet the mechanism was invisible. He likened it to the force the moon exerts on our planet's water causing unfailingly regular tides, or the invisible force which causes a magnet to attract iron shavings in predictable patterns. The forces themselves could not be seen in his time, but the tides could be predicted with great precision. These forces still cannot be seen in our time, and perhaps never will be; but very few people seriously question whether they exist. We know them by the effects they have in the world, which are indeed visible and measurable.

The method Hahnemann invented for the preparation of remedies involves repeated dilution of the medicinal substance. But between dilutions the solution must be subjected to forceful agitation. This is performed in a specified way, and a specified number of times, to give consistent results. Making a remedy is a long, careful process. The more times a remedy is put throught this whole sequence, the higher its potency.

We're accustomed to assuming that a larger amount of something is a stronger agent of change; and on the scale of regular, chemical drugs, that's generally true (but remember the principle of hormesis which shows the opposite is true at certain scales). It can be confusing at first that at the energetic level, the greater the dilution, the higher the potency.

In a similar way, we feel sure furniture, mountains, and our bodies are made of solid matter—while the foundational theories of modern science have been telling us for more than two hundred years that isn't the case at all. Our absolute belief in a world of solid matter is a result of the natural limits of our perception. Interestingly, modern atomic theory developed in parallel with homeopathy. Perhaps humanity was just becoming ready to understand its world—and itself—in a new, more subtle way.

In most homeopathic potencies, there are no ordinary molecules of the original substance. But nanoparticles remain, and as the potency rises, they begin to form clusters, and increasingly large, complex structures.[29] A homeopathic remedy introduces the material's energetic "signature" into an organism. The energy fields which govern its life permeate every part of the organism, so it is not necessary to target an organ, tissue, or chemical pathway, or introduce large quantities of medication.

Since the early twentieth century other discoveries in biology and chemistry have also helped to illuminate the way the remedies may interact with our physiological processes. The advances in mainstream science are bound to be as important to understanding the action of the remedies as studies focused on the remedies themselves. Scientists working in water research have made discoveries which are revolutionizing biology. (Slowly—because, again, the more radical and paradigm-shaking a discovery is, the greater the opposition it encounters.) In brief, there is a fourth state of water: aside from the vapor, liquid and frozen states, water often exists in a highly structured, gel-like form.[30,31]

Water inside and around our cells, it has been found, is typically in this fourth phase. Information and energy are stored and transmitted through this medium. Prominent individuals in biology, chemistry, physics, medicine, technology, agriculture, and other professions form an international community which continues to investigate this critical topic. Their findings have led some of them to speak out publicly on behalf of homeopathy's plausibility.

The remedies are being investigated in other ways as well. At a molecular biology lab in the UK, scientists have been analyzing potencies using solvatochromic dyes in many different experiments since 2009.[32] The results consistently show that potentized solutions behave differently from unpotentized solutions. Each remedy displays unique characteristics, and the presence of the remedy produces a "polarizing and structuring effect" on the solution. The group has experimented with the application of a weak electric current to the remedy solution, simulating the electrical environment within a living organism. After a brief, predictable delay, the solution begins to emit photons.[33] In other words, at a very subtle scale, it begins to glow. Plain water does not do this!

A hypothesis has been proposed regarding the spin of electrons. It suggests that the mechanism of the disturbance of human energy fields is a reversal in the spin of electrons.[34] Such a reversal has been shown to occur when atoms are exposed to electromagnetic influences. This could help to explain both the loss of stability in human energy fields following injury, stress, or shock, and the restorative effects of a correctly chosen homeopathic remedy.

The mitochondria in living cells perform many complex functions, far beyond the energy production and storage described in our high school biology textbooks. They organize in vast numbers, changing their shapes, migrating great distances, congregating in organized formations, coordinating activities, engaging in communication both within and between cells.[35] One of their confirmed functions is mediating epigenetic changes in our DNA.[36] It is also known that mitochondria interact with light. Sophisticated biophoton therapies are being developed in conventional medicine. A 2021 study at the University of Johannesburg determined that both photodynamic therapy and homeopathic treatment could induce self-destruction (apoptosis) of cancer cells.[37]

A professor at Strasbourg University spent many years studying the interface of biology, chemistry, and quantum physics. He proposed a mechanism of action of homeopathic potencies based on the well-established phenomenon of entanglement and other aspects of quantum field theory. He remarks: "Time is now ripe for physicians and biologists to realise that quantum physics applies at all scales, giving homeopathy its credentials as a rational medical approach for healing people."[38] This message is encountered again and again from physicists who have made a serious study of the homeopathy question.

Many others are also pursuing quantum field theory approaches, incorporating highly creative thinking and innovative study models.[39] Quantum electrodynamics provides a durable model of health and disease based on the coherence of electromagnetic fields in living organisms.[40] Energy moves in waves through electromagnetic fields, and disruption of these waves results in measurable loss of healthy physiological function.

This model may also help to explain the transfer of information through water within organisms—which we now realize is water in its highly orginized, liquid crystalline, or gel-like, state. Energy medicine, such as homeopathy, can reorganize and regulate energy fields. In the coming decades, research in this area will change medicine profoundly.

Perhaps the largest area of research—or the area in which the other avenues converge—is that of homeopathic remedies as nanomedicines. The presence of nanoparticles of the original medicinal substance in potentized solutions has been repeatedly confirmed by at least a dozen research centers worldwide. Nanomedicine is already embraced in medical research and practice as an incredibly valuable approach to non-invasive healing. Cutting edge conventional medicine is increasingly oriented toward subtler, safer, more individualized and targeted therapies. Cooperation between homeopathic and conventional researchers and physicians should flourish in the years ahead.

The universe is full of phenomena that we observe with wonder and can't immediately understand. The seemingly mysterious effectiveness of homeopathy was one of them, but the benefit people experienced provided ample momentum to sustain its practice. Homeopathy was once seen as highly improbable, but that is no longer the case for those who are informed. It's a beautiful example of the self-correcting property of science: the very fields which once were thought to contradict homeopathy are now at the forefront in its validation.

The practical need for a holistic view of health is more universally accepted every year. Just as Hahnemann's controversial ideas about mental health, diet, personal hygiene, and hereditary factors in disease now seem obvious, the tenets of holistic healthcare are being integrated into mainstream medicine and into public consciousness. These include the direct physiological impact of stress and trauma; the individualized ways we respond to pathogens, life experiences, environmental factors, and medicines; the critical role of our inner "terrain" in disease prevention and recovery; and the tremendous power of epigenetics for degeneration or regeneration.

# 8
# Why is homeopathy controversial?

Back in Hahnemann's time, homeopathy provoked resentment, derision, and even outrage. There are still aggressive critics today. Interestingly, the harangues, and the hostility behind them, have not essentially changed over the last two centuries. Some continue to repeat misinformation about homeopathy, year after year, stubbornly refusing to fairly assess—or even acknowledge—the massive amount of data.

A handful of individuals have enjoyed making a public entertainment out of "debunking" homeopathy. They assert that it is "anti-science" while deliberately ignoring the abundant, readily available research. Is that a scientific approach? If you listen closely, you will notice they don't substantiate their claims against classical homeopathy, justify their accusations that homeopaths are charlatans, or address the evidence for homeopathy. Some liken it to a magic trick—a comparison which is in very poor taste, to put it mildly. Medicine is not a joke when you're coping with illness. Nor is it amusing that most people consult a homeopath only after surviving years of disappointment or outright damage from conventional medicine.

It makes little sense to criticize something you don't understand, or even try to understand. One wonders why people who profess to care about public health insist on maintaining a status quo in which millions of people suffer without hope. Many people are as afraid of medical treatments as they are of life-threatening disease. What do these pseudoskeptics gain by their malicious conduct? While sincere skepticism is vitally important in science, unthinking dogmatism obstructs learning, healthy questioning, and genuine progress.

Homeopathy is sometimes characterized by detractors as a "fringe" modality. The direct experience of billions of people, over many generations, is far too powerful a testimony to be so casually dismissed. Homeopathy is not more improbable than many other natural phenomena accepted by modern science. Nor is it stranger than many of today's state-of-the-art technologies, including highly successful nanomedicines, diagnostic imaging, and other accepted (and rightly celebrated) advances. High-quality science supports the premises these technologies share with energy medicine.

The most controversial aspect of homeopathy has been the use of extreme dilutions. Conventional medicine confines itself within strict biochemical parameters, and this is fine. But insisting that its model is the only valid or useful way of working with human health is simply foolish, and is detrimental to the public good.

There is no reason homeopathy should not be viewed through a lens of respect, curiosity, and cooperation. And so it is, in most parts of the world; oddly, it's the English-speaking nations that lag behind. One compelling reason it is worthy of esteem is that it has always been driven by the wish to help people heal, not by desire for profit or power. It holds the trust of many millions of people, not because all those millions are unintelligent or delusional (as some critics have publicly stated) but because it does, in fact, help people become well and stay well.

Among many other positive outcomes, greater access to holistic care could relieve—or perhaps *rescue* is a better word—our overwhelmed and dysfunctional medical services. The disdain of the ignorant has never made homeopathy go away, and it never will. But the longer its general acceptance is delayed, the more people will suffer unnecessarily.

Important discoveries always begin with observing surprising, inexplicable phenomena. Often we accept and use them in practical ways for many years—or even for many centuries—before we decipher how they work. This is the natural order of the scientific process. To give one conspicuous example, we know that the law of gravity impacts the entire universe; yet the world's top experts in physics still don't have even a tentative notion of what it is, where it comes from, why or how it operates as it does. We still do exactly as Hahnemann did in 1800: observe and measure a natural force by its effects on its surroundings.

Throughout the history of science, from ancient times to the present, the more important a discovery is, the more adjustment it requires in the way we think about things—and the way we manufacture, regulate, and sell things—and therefore, the more hostility it meets. Not so long ago, earnest and brilliant scientists were exiled, imprisoned, even executed for proposing ideas that threatened the status quo , such as the preposterous claim that the Earth is not the center of the universe!

Classical homeopaths (and others in alternative med-icine) fully understand that there are times when the modality they practice is not the appropriate one. Any responsible practitioner will refer to another kind of care, including conventional medical care, when that is the best course of action for the person who is ill. Many are happy to integrate their skills with the work of others. The widespread reluctance or refusal of medical doctors to do the same is odd, to say the least.

One reason, then, that homeopathy is controversial is that it takes a long time for science and society to make major adjustments to their understanding. But there is another reason: there are some serious conflicts *within* homeopathy. Usually introductory books refrain from addressing this. It does require more thoughtfulness on the part of the reader, but I believe anyone who is considering using homeopathy needs to be candidly informed.

Some homeopaths sustain the rational approach established by Hahnemann. Others prefer to rely on subjective notions to choose a remedy. Some of the objections to homeopathy are exacerbated by methods of practice which are not only ungrounded in science, but have abandoned the foundational principles which have always made homeopathy reliable and safe. The different types of homeopathic practice, and how to recognize and choose one that is right for you, will be discussed in Chapter Eleven.

# 9
# Is it true that homeopathy is a placebo?

You will sometimes hear people say that homeopathy acts only as a placebo. With just a little thought, it's clear that this is incorrect. The preceding chapters have introduced, in simplified form, the theory and science which underlie homeopathic practice. The placebo effect is a very interesting and important phenomenon in medicine of any kind, and a brief discussion of it may be useful.

Our beliefs can alter our perceptions, and can even induce physiological changes. People often feel better in significant ways after consulting any kind of trusted practitioner. The placebo effect is not limited to medical situations though; a person may feel energized, or find physical discomforts improved, after being with a beloved friend, receiving good news, or visiting a place that has spiritual significance to them. The benefit is real and welcome. It shows that the healing force has been stimulated and has created movement within the organism in the direction of well being.

Placebo effects in the context of medication and drug studies are well known. Placebo surgeries have been very successful in the treatment of serious internal and joint conditions. Up to 75 percent of medical doctors give a placebo or non-specific therapy at least once a week. (A non-specific therapy is an actual intervention, but one which is not indicated for the problem at hand—antibiotics for a viral infection, or blood tests or imaging that have no use in the situation.) This amounts to giving a placebo in many cases, since its only purpose is to reassure a patient that something is being done for them.

The most pronounced placebo effects tend to be in pain relief and the sense of well-being. Being a "placebo responder" has generally been seen in the medical world as a negative trait of certain people. But why? Surely the sensitivity and readiness of an organism to create healing change are very positive.

The placebo effect does not happen only to certain people. There is no way to know beforehand who will experience a placebo response, because a natural healing process can occur in any living organism. But not all disease conditions respond to placebos. Infections and cancerous tumors for example are not altered, even if the person temporarily feels better. If homeopathy was simply a placebo, it obviously would not have the track record it does: bringing healing or cure to deep and dif-ficult pathologies for 230 years. Is every case cured? Of course not. That is the reality in any medical system. All treatments are chosen and administered by human beings, who are fallible, and treatment is only one of many variables in any given case.

When a correct homeopathic remedy is given, there is a specific pattern of response. It can continue to evolve over long periods of time, requiring careful long-term monitoring. This is a complex subject (students at good homeopathic colleges spend many months learning about it) but for our purposes in this book, it is sufficient to say that the course of improvement seen with proper homeopathic care is very different from what is seen with the placebo effect. We know that improvement from a placebo is neither predictable nor durable, while response to homeopathic treatment can be both. A mild, temporary aggravation of one or more symptoms is expected following a correct remedy (in fact it's an important sign); this is absent with placebos.

Based on natural laws governing all living organisms, homeopathy is effective for animals and plants as well as people. It is equally useful for infants and children, adults, pets, livestock, farms and orchards, gardens, and beehives. There have been homeopathic veterinarians for two hundred years. I am personally acquainted with several homeopaths who undertook years of study and career change in midlife because they were so impressed with the healing they saw in their pets after working with a homeopathic veterinarian.

Agrohomeopathy, using the remedies in the context of farming and gardening, is a more recent development. Its use is growing rapidly, because it is often more effective, always more affordable, and unquestionably safer than industrial chemicals. Nutrient deficiencies, depleted or contaminated soil, weather damage, insect infestations, and fungal, viral and bacterial diseases are being prevented, managed, or cured.

Using agrohomeopathy, one is freed from one of the huge problems created by pesticides, resistant pests, as using homeopathy for people and animals with infections rather than antibiotics (in appropriate cases) can help resolve the dreadful dilemma of antibiotic- and anti-viral resistant pathogens. Industrial agriculture is environmentally destructive and terribly expensive, perpetuating a grim economic divide. It is totally reliant on fossil fuels and its final product is nutrient-poor and contaminated. This model of agriculture is one of the most significant drivers of climate disaster on local and global scales. As an affordable, non-toxic alternative to myriad agricultural problems, agro-homeopathy is one of the most important (and, so far, least appreciated) breakthroughs of our time. It's absolutely clear that this gathering revolution is not based on placebo response.

Classical homeopathy is not based on hope of placebo effect or on miracle cures. As one of the most important homeopathic doctors, J. T. Kent, remarked, homeopathy is not guesswork or wishful thinking but an applied science. The placebo effect is based on knowledge and belief about being sick, and also beliefs about taking medicine. It is obvious that infants and small children, people with cognitive disabilities, people who are unconscious, cats and dogs and rabbits and chickens, apple trees, rows of crops, communities of honey bees, and soil microorganisms are not manifesting placebo effects. Nor are the millions of people who daily heal and recover from the use of properly practiced homeopathic medicine.

# 10
# I tried a remedy and it didn't work. Why?

Homeopathic remedy selection is a very different process from using the more familiar over-the-counter or prescription medications. For a remedy to improve your health, it must be correctly matched not to one symptom or to a diagnosis, but to the complete picture of what's occuring in you, as a whole organism. This includes your mental and emotional state, symptoms associated with the current illness, and details of all sorts such as temperature regulation, sleep patterns, reactions to climate and foods, and much more.

The remedies that are sold in stores usually have a label which says "headache," "insomnia," or something similar, but only because the FDA requires an indication on the label. There are hundreds of remedies which might be indicated for headache or insomnia. If you have chronic or recurring headaches or insomnia, the chances of that one in the shop being the correct one for you are actually quite small.

A professional homeopath has a reference library, cross-referenced computer programs, years of training, and a worldwide community of colleagues to help them make the right choice. The reference materials have been compiled over more than two centuries, and they are infamously perplexing. They contain a huge amount of information, much of it in obsolete language, and without adequate preparation they seem to be full of contradictions. Over the years more has been added, but little subtracted; some dedicated souls have given their time to bring greater organization to it all, but it remains challenging to say the least. For the beginner, the references may provoke more questions than they answer.

Additionally, every remedy is available in a wide range of potencies. Even assuming you have the correct remedy, an unsuitable potency will not have the desired effect, if it has any effect at all. It takes some finesse to correctly judge the best potency in a given case. The number and schedule of doses will certainly effect the outcome. Often it is necessary to switch to a different remedy as the situation changes, which starts the whole selection process over again. You can see that choosing a remedy from a label on a vial, a self-help book, or a brief online primer course is not likely to consistently give good results. The medicines are called remedies, but this doesn't mean they are "home remedies" in the sense of being simple and straightforward for everyone to use at home.

All of that being said, there are certain situations in which home treatment may work well. There are kits containing commonly used remedies for acutes such as the common cold or flu, minor burns, or food poisoning. Using these together with a good manual can be quite satisfactory. There are excellent kits designed for travel, pregnancy, birth, and the care of young children or pets. These can be used when the conditions you treat are truly self-limiting.

A few schools offer good courses designed for those who want to provide basic healthcare for themselves and their families. Be cautious about short courses that promise to make you proficient in homeopathy in a few weeks. It may be founded on elegantly simple principles, but treating living beings, in real-world situations, is a skill that develops neither quickly nor easily. Also, as practitioners of all kinds know, objectively assessing the symptoms of people you are close to (or your own symptoms) is especially tricky.

Frequently, self-prescribing results in frustration, and in this scenario people sometimes decide that "homeopathy doesn't work for me." This is very unfortunate, because they will miss out on a lifetime of profound benefit from proper homeopathic care. Naturally, just as in conventional medicine or any other kind of treatment, if you take the wrong prescription it will not solve your problem. That doesn't mean the medicine is defective, or that your condition wouldn't respond well to the right medicine. The idea that homeopathy only works for some people is another common misconception.

What if you have been working with a professional homeopath and have not experienced progress? There are many reasons this could occur. It's possible that the homeopath has not understood the nature of your problem. Clearly communicating all the relevant details to them can be challenging for some people. But it's also possible that your condition is complex and will take time and patient effort to resolve. No matter what kind of healthcare we choose, the progress we make toward good health will depend on many factors: our heredity, living circumstances and lifestyle, past medical treatments, our stress level, and more.

A concern many homeopaths express is that sometimes people expect dramatic improvements after a very short time, or after taking just one remedy. Such expectations are likely to lead to disappointment. "Why,"

I heard a homeopath lament, "has my client given the medical system twenty-five years to try to help her, has taken their medication every day for years, but only gave me a month and has given up on homeopathy?" Similarly, people may accept without question that for even a moderate injury, they may need to attend physical therapy several times a week for months, but when trying homeopathy for the first time, they might feel disillusioned if they don't experience immediate relief. Both becoming sick and becoming well are processes. Cells, organs, and the body's chemical systems may take time to heal. True health is worth the investment of some patience.

Another possible reason for lack of progress is that not all homeopaths observe the guiding principles of homeopathy, and alternative methodologies can yield inconsistent results. If you want to work with a homeopath, it's important to realize that different people practice in very different ways. It is well worth taking the time to make sure you find someone whose methods seem right to you. In Chapter Eleven we will look more closely at some different types of homeopathy.

For a serious or chronic condition it's essential not to try to design your own homeopathic treatment. Learn to keep firmly in mind that all aspects of a person are interconnected. Chronic problems which seem minor or ordinary are actually part of a much bigger pattern which can best be seen by a trained eye. To name a few examples, recurring migraines, menstrual problems, allergies, mood swings, skin conditions, blood sugar troubles, and repeated infections are experienced by so many people these days that they may be seen as "normal." But a recurring or chronic problem is always a sign that an underlying disturbance exists.

Experimenting and taking incorrect remedies can make your symptoms more confusing and delay healing. Homeopathy is not a folk remedy, nor is it so easily learned as the use of herbs. It's a sophisticated system of healthcare which requires years of dedication to master, just like any other highly skilled profession.

Finally, there are many combination remedy products available to the general public now, beautifully packaged and skillfully marketed. They target particular symptoms or syndromes: allergies, arthritis, anxiety, indigestion, and so on. They might seem to be the perfect compromise: you get to use natural medicine, in magic bullet form. But as you now know, a remedy must be chosen for the whole person. The reasons for avoiding combinations will become clearer in the next chapter.

# 11
# How should I choose a homeopath?

When you are unwell, what you need to know is: will this person be able to help me? Or when your child is sick: will this treatment be safe? Will it help them heal or set them back? Homeopaths practice in very different ways. And as patients or clients we may be looking for different kinds of consultation or intervention. How can you choose a practitioner who is right for you?

I will begin by saying that my understanding and practice are aligned firmly with classical homeopathy. But for years, that was not the case. Like many, I was hungry for ideas and I encountered ideas, more or less at random, which seemed fascinating. I didn't have a foundational comprehension of homeopathy (though I thought I did!), so I could not realistically evaluate those ideas. I did what so many do: I attempted to build something with all the interesting pieces.

The truth I had to admit, quite soon, was that the sum of those pieces did not permit a coherent practice. I did my best to help myself and others. The real problem wasn't that the results were not always as good as I hoped; every practitioner wishes for complete cure every time, which is not possible. The key problem, I realized, was that the results were *totally unpredictable.* I felt that should never be the case in a medical system, although I saw that some homeopaths seemed resigned to it. My disillusionment was deep and painful. But I had myself experienced the profound changes a right remedy could stimulate. I could not give up on homeopathy.

Over the years I attended several schools teaching very different philosophies and methods. I've done many seminars from yet other schools, and read and conversed widely. My own point of view changed a great deal over the years. But its evolution was not only due to all the schooling. It was also informed by long years as a patient with serious health challenges of my own—and as a parent. Some very vital lessons have been learned from the other side of the desk.

While writing this book, I asked non-classical homeopaths for their feedback, and reflected on my own thoughts in the early years. I have tried to understand and communicate various points of view. I'm sure the result is neither complete nor perfect; however, I believe the following discussion can ignite your own thinking, wondering, and questioning. And that is the true purpose of this chapter (and this book).

The first piece which must be in place is to know what you are looking for when you begin your search. This chapter will explore some of the important variations. Almost all homeopaths will be happy to talk with you about their practice, and will do their best to answer your questions. They know that trying a new kind of healthcare is an important and courageous step. They are, in my experience, universally passionate about their work, and care deeply about helping people.

Now there are once again homeopathic colleges in the United States and Canada, and thanks to the internet, some people attend international schools. But in most parts of North America homeopathy is an unregulated profession. This means a homeopath (except in Ontario and Arizona, as of this writing) cannot be licensed as a medical professional, no matter how much education or experience they have. It also means that there are no government-approved standards for education and practice.

There are professional organizations which strive to provide educational, ethical, and theoretical standards. The Council for Homeopathic Certification, for example, allows people to use the designation Certified

Classical Homeopath (CCH) after passing examinations and submitting a certain number of successfully treated cases. Confusingly, though, some people become a CCH because it lends credibility, but then practice non-classical styles of homeopathy.

Because there were no formal education options for several generations, homeopaths generally learned through years of independent study, apprenticeship, and mentoring. Many still do, or they combine formal and traditional methods of learning. Herbalists and midwives are still sometimes educated through apprenticeship as well. This was true in conventional medicine too, for centuries, and in some ways today's period of residency following medical school preserves the tradition.

Financial aid, scholarships, and tax credits, supports taken for granted in most fields of study, are virtually non-existent for the students of homeopathic colleges. Many people become homeopaths later in life, after other degrees and careers, while raising families, and often after facing life-changing illness in themselves or their children. The financial and scheduling demands of formal education are simply not possible for some, or they must complete their schooling in stages over a longer time while fulfilling other commitments. Though they may lack the honorifics, these individuals sometimes bring a unique richness of experience to their practice.

While there are many philosophies and methods, the essential differences can be roughly understood in terms of classical versus non-classical homeopathy. In other words, does the homeopath practice according to the four essential principles discussed earlier in this book? We will consider why that question is so important.

There are too many new variations on the theme of homeopathy to even mention here. In fact, there are virtually unlimited variations, because without the framework of the basic principles, each homeopath can do whatever they choose. Some even practice differently from one day to the next. Others work consistently, in accordance with newer theoretical systems. Different methods can produce radically different outcomes.

Please do not be put off if this seems perplexing. Homeopathy, well used, has tremendous positive potential for every one of us, and it is well worth pondering these questions at the beginning. You will see that with an understanding of the basics, you will have no trouble choosing who you want to work with.

The following section will revisit the foundational principles of homeopathy, explaining how contemporary homeopaths sometimes depart from them, and some of the implications of those departures. Then there will be a discussion of the remedies themselves; some new remedies have been introduced whose reliability is debated.

The law of similars is probably the most widely agreed upon point—at least in theory. The question is, how does a homeopath discern which remedy is most similar, if not through the established process described in the previous chapters? One newer approach attributes symbolic meanings to people's vocabulary, appearance, and gestures. Sometimes remedies are selected based on an imaginative impulse ("He suddenly reminded me of a..."). Sometimes the challenge is avoided altogether by giving many remedies all at once.

According to one doctrine, patients unconsciously communicate which remedy they need by using keywords in their speech (such as "incomplete" or "caught"). How are these abstractions translated into a remedy? The words are matched with a chart created by individuals who believe they can interpret or channel the subjective inner experiences of plants, animals, and even minerals, and have assigned keywords to them.

This style, known as the Sensation Method, includes a multitude of categories, diagrams, and theoretical structures, cobbling together a host of speculative notions. In fact these many moving parts can be contradictory, and no effort is made toward objective confirmation. People who like this collage of ideas simply agree to regard it as a legitimate method.

A related practice relies on choosing a remedy based on the "kingdom" which the homeopath believes corresponds to the person. For example, a woman attends her first consultation wearing a colorful, flowery dress. Among her complaints are allergies and sensitivity to noise. She will be considered a "plant" person, and the practitioner will only consider remedies made from plants for her. Someone who wears understated clothes and works in finance must be given a mineral remedy; a person who is highly competitive needs an animal-based remedy, and so on.

There is heated debate: does this method reflect the individuality of the patient, or unfounded assumptions on the part of the homeopath? (And what on Earth should be done with a client who likes flowers *and* pinstripes? Perhaps yesterday that "plant" woman wore a grey suit.)

Some classify remedies according to their position in the Periodic Table of Elements. A symbolic philosophy has been introduced which postulates that the stages of development of a human being, and of humanity in general, correspond to the physical properties of the elements. The theory is elegant and well-developed, and has a devoted following.

In fact, many of the chemical elements have undergone extensive provings and have been used since the early days of homeopathy. Their characteristics have accumulated an enormous amount of confirmation, which often aligns very well with the Periodic Table theory. Other elements, however, have not been proved, but are prescribed according to the qualities they are *presumed* to have, based on their position in the table. There is disagreement about whether this degree of extrapolation is acceptable in a medical setting.

There are many other ideas which may influence remedy selection, but this gives you a snapshot of a few of the more common trends. They vary widely in the rationality of their concepts and the reliability of their results. The lack of standardized oversight in homeopathy can be troubling in this context. A practitioner may say their client is "better." But for how long are they better? When some symptoms are better, do others begin to appear? There *are* reliable, practical ways of evaluating long-term progress, but many homeopaths do not use them or even know about them.

Some contemporary practitioners work from extensive classical training, but feel one of the new methods (or aspects of it) is an important innovation. Others blend several, untroubled by the fact that the various theories lead to contradictory conclusions, or they may improvise as they go through each consultation. Some choose the remedy based on a momentary impulse they believe is given to them by a higher power, or employ divination techniques when they are unsure which remedy to choose.

From the point of view of many classical homeopaths, there are concerning flaws in these new methods. Some ask, for example: How can we presume to know the inner experience, the "vital sensation," of a tree, an invertebrate, or a metal? Why would we approach the task that way, adding layers of subjectivity and guesswork, rather than focus on what is clear and present? Is it within the purview of a healthcare practitioner to attribute anthropomorphic feelings such as "downtrodden" or "trapped," or sensations such as "suffocating," to inanimate materials, molluscs, flowers, insects, bacteria, and use this as a basis for medical prescription?

Is it acceptable to rely on preconceived notions about a person's inner nature, or their disease state, based on their language, gestures, the subject they studied in college, their jewelry or hairstyle? The subjective experience of the client is of paramount importance in homeopathy. It is a foundational rule, however, that the homeopath must strive to be as unprejudiced as possible in order to see and hear the patient's experience clearly. How is inserting people into clever but artificial categories reconciled with the fundamental principle that we are all unique individuals?

If the premises are acceptable, how does one manage all the variables? What about cultural differences in demeanor? These are so real that peoples have literally gone to war over misunderstood gestures. Words and phrases are used differently by non-native speakers; language habits are formed by families and communities; clothing might have more to do with a person's budget or social situation than their soul, ideology, or inherent psychological disposition. What about the undeniable fact that plant remedies have the qualities which allegedly belong to minerals, and vice versa? Competitiveness is seen as "animal," but no gardener is ignorant of the fact that plants can be competitive. And do animal and plant tissues not also contain minerals?

In short, what if the sensations attributed to various materials are not a revealed truth, but rather a runaway anthropormorphic abstraction? What if the Kingdom Method is likewise baseless? Just how many "what ifs" are allowable in a medical profession? Unfortunately, when I have tried to open these questions with contemporary practitioners, they have usually been shrugged off, or are met with a highly defensive attitude. If these ideas are valid, and if helping a sick person to heal is the true aim, candid discussion is necessary.

Some of the newer philosophies may be compelling; pondering or discussing the ideas they raise might (or might not) be interesting and worthwhile. The relevant question, however, for most people seeking healthcare alternatives, is whether they provide a sufficient basis for giving real medicines to real people with real illness.

There is a crucial difference between intuition and imagination. Losing sight of this difference may be at the heart of some of the misunderstandings in homeopathy today. Intuition is a type of direct perception; imagination refers to constructs our minds create by connecting fragments of information (fragments which may be factual, or may come from something we saw, heard, assumed or dreamed). There isn't necessarily any connection between them outside of our own thoughts.

A helpful example of an imaginative assumption is the starry constellations we recognize in the sky. The stars, for instance, in the constellation called Orion are not, in physical reality, associated with each other as our learned tradition tells us they are. They are only related from our subjective point of view, which does not register the vast distances between them (in both space and time). Our imagination creates a strangely convincing two-dimensional picture from a few points of light. The Hunter is not there except in our cultural imaginative consensus, and yet as soon as we're taught to recognize him, we can't help seeing him. In other cultures, the same stars are just as indelibly associated with a hand, a deer, a canoe. Might this confusion between imagination and intuition help to explain the tangential course contemporary homeopathy has taken?

In artistic and other creative contexts, imagination has purpose and meaning. In a medical setting, the needs and expectations are different. But most (if not all) great leaps in science have been founded on intuitive insights. How do we know whether something true and important has occured to us through such an insight, or whether we're believing—maybe even ready to fight to defend—an imaginary construct, perhaps one totally incompatible with the circumstances? To what extent has ego intruded? Because this is such a very tricky matter, humans have always made efforts to question, compare, experiment, verify. We call that process science. One could say that science, in this context, means caring enough to make sure. We need our practitioners to ask themselves, are they making the best effort they can to understand what they are doing, and why?

There is a rift in homeopathy regarding the principle of the single remedy. Some contemporary practitioners have said that due to the complexity of modern health problems, one remedy at a time is no longer sufficient. They believe classical homeopathy is too rigid on this point and is needlessly restrictive. To this, classical homeopaths counter that with increasingly difficult disease states, it is all the more important to be clear and careful. The rule, they say, is based on observable, verifiable properties of nature, which do not expire and cannot be outdated. How exactly does mixing remedies improve treatment? This question too still awaits a clear answer from its proponents.

To understand why classical homeopaths are adamant about the rule of the single remedy, recall the idea of resonance, discussed in Chapter Six. Imagine a tuning fork is sounding one steady frequency. How can several different frequencies be the one which resonates with it to create the same pitch? Obviously this is not possible. Even if one of the remedies is a good match, wouldn't others given at the same time interfere? How could the result not be a confusing dissonance?

The rule of the single remedy is not preserved out of sentimental attachment to "old ways," nor out of a stubborn or dogmatic mindset. It is maintained because combinations of remedies can *increase* the disorder within an already struggling organism. When multiple remedies are taken, especially high potencies or many doses, there will undoubtedly be changes, but change does not equal healing. Physical symptoms may morph into new problems, possibly shifting to a more vital level. In other words, they may be replaced by emotional, cognitive, or psychological symptoms which are unlikely to be immediately visible. Combining remedies (known as *pluralism*) brings us right back to the world of side effects, suppression, and confusion.

How can we interpret the response of the vital force when it has received multiple discordant stimulations? Which remedies are causing the changes? Are several remedies reacting with each other, and with the vital energy? Is the disease becoming more serious, while its natural expressions are obscured?

When the resulting confusion is hastily treated with yet more combinations, soon any hope of observing the evolution of the disease, or the efforts of the vital force, is lost. A person who came seeking better health now may be in diminishing health. I am very sorry to say that I have seen individuals whose psychological and physical health have become hopelessly deranged in this way. The damage can eventually become virtually impossible to unravel. To my knowledge, there has never been a single proving or other study of a combination remedy, which raises massive practical and ethical questions.

The principle of individualized prescribing is again ostensibly accepted by almost all homeopaths. But questions again arise about pluralism. It cannot be called individualized; the prescription is not based on the unique corresponding patterns of the patient and the remedy. In fact, technically, it is not homeopathy at all. If this is the style of practice, it should be overtly acknowledged that it is not the medical system known for centuries as homeopathy. I believe it needs to find a name of its own to resolve the great confusion we see today. As more states and provinces regulate homeopathic practice (and they will), hopefully clearer definitions and boundaries will be established.

The principle of the minimum dose states that we should use the smallest dose which is effective, because it has been abundantly proven that this stimulates the natural healing capacity best. This would mean the lowest effective potency, and the smallest effective number of doses. But how do we know how much is effective? Centuries of combined experience and analysis, have laid out some rational guidelines. To this must be added practical experience and finely tuned evaluative skills. The law of the minimum effective dose is consistent with universal ideas of medical ethics. Sometimes this means only one dose. Reality is nuanced, however, and many details about each individual and their ongoing circumstances must be considered. It is not something that can ever be completely standardized. The natural law of individuality is always with us.

The question of safety arises in connection with this rule. There are some who believe that if the remedy does not resonate *exactly* with the vital energy, it will have no effect. Some claim that homeopathic remedies are always safe, no matter which one you use, or how many you use, or what potency, or how often. But how could that be true? If a substance has the capacity to stimulate change, we cannot assume it will only stimulate changes we like. Homeopathy was invented, after all, to move medicine away from indiscriminate and overbearing interventions.

With reasonable, knowledgeable use of the remedies, they are extremely safe—one could argue they are the safest of all human medicines, more harmless than herbs or even many foods. The rule of the minimum dose always allows repetition of a remedy as needed, or increasing the potency as indicated. It permits the use of high potencies when there is a basis for doing so.

Regenerating cells and tissues, resolving pathological conditions, takes time. After all, it took a period of time for the damage to occur; chronic or severe disease states are usually the result of many years of disturbance. No homeopath or doctor will make something heal faster than the natural healing process can heal it. It should hardly be surprising that erratic, incorrect, or excessive use of any kind of medicine can cause problems.

The minimum dose rule reminds us to be guided by the organism's response to the medicine. If we don't wait long enough to observe the organism's response, how can we proceed intelligently? We can't know whether the remedy was correct, whether it has stimulated the healing process, or whether that stimulation was strong enough, unless we allow the vital force time to work. If the remedy is right, why would it be necessary to give an excessive amount? Reckless dosing or repetition shows an apparent lack of trust in the natural healing process. Some practitioners seem to forget that homeopathy's role is to support that natural process, not to force change.

Too large and frequent doses amount to a flood of energetic impulses. The problem is compounded by doing this with multiple remedies. What chaos this must introduce into an organism which is already stressed—and how much more complicated the situation becomes! Not only our physical health, but our mental balance, our sense of who we are and how we relate to the world around us, emerge from the underlying energetic level of our lives. Drastic overstimulation at that level has the potential to be profoundly destabilizing. These interactions must not continue to be ignored or dismissed.

Note that when the situation is acute more frequent doses may be needed. With an infection or an injury, during childbirth, or in palliative care (a situation in which homeopathy shines) the picture may evolve quickly. With rapid or sudden onset of symptoms, the whole process may be accelerated, including recovery. In such a case, a sequence of doses may be needed in a relatively short time.

A final topic to touch on regarding philosophical and practical differences in homeopathic practice is that of provings. Are all of the remedies equally reliable and well-studied? In fact their properties range from deeply and thoroughly understood to virtually unknown.

The original remedies were proved through the rigorous methods laid out by Hahnemann. But, perhaps surprisingly, modern provings have rarely followed that method faithfully. Now, many virtually unstudied remedies are available, inducing disagreement among homeopaths, as well as drawing criticism from outside the homeopathic community. Is a complete traditional proving important?

The idea of individuality—that we each have a unique set of sensitivities—is central to homeopathy. Though it may not be obvious at first glance, it's also central to the proving process. The foundational first step of a classical proving is to assemble a group of *suitable* provers. To do this, the new remedy is administered to a group of people. But only a minority of those people will be sensitive to it (if any). Only those who definitely react to it can be used as provers. The rest clearly cannot give a meaningful proving of the remedy, because they are not responsive to it and will not express its symptoms.

This first round is unlikely to yield a sufficient number of provers, in which case the process must be repeated with new volunteers, as many times as necessary to assemble a large enough group that you can conduct an effective study. It can take a relatively long time to collect this group; but having done so, you begin the proving knowing that every prover's symptoms will be valid and useful.

However, most modern provings have omitted this first phase. Instead, the proving is conducted with any group that is convenient, such as a class at a homeopathy school. There is a certain prestige associated with conducting provings and introducing new remedies, and of course they generate books and seminars. Some people have put an enormous amount of time and effort into provings, following the rest of Hahnemann's steps, but using a group that has not be screened to make sure they actually respond to the remedy. It is reasonable, then, to ask: how can we be sure that the results are reliable?

Some of the observations those volunteers report may be due to the remedy; but logic tells us that many of them can't be. From the massive amount of information gathered, there is no way to know which are valid indications about the remedy and which are simply changes that people noticed some time after the dose. We know that the power of suggestion can prompt changes or increase people's awareness of them (this is one reason classical provings include a control group which unknowingly receives a placebo).

Some are concerned that through these incomplete provings, remedies are coming into use which we don't understand as well as we should. The data associated with them inevitably includes a significant amount of erroneous information. But those "symptoms" will be included in new editions of some reference books, and thereafter accepted as fact. Patients, of course, and even many contemporary homeopaths, do not know which remedies have been thoroughly researched and which have not.

Sometimes at a weekend seminar the attendees are given a vial with an unknown remedy in it. They keep the vial with them throughout the seminar. On the final day, people report any changes, symptoms, or unusual impressions experienced during the weekend. Sensations, emotions, dreams are noted and analyzed, looking for patterns.

No one has ingested—or even touched—the remedy in this scenario. All the participants are away from home attending an intense and costly event, surrounded by strangers, often in a foreign country, eating unfamiliar food and suddenly immersed in a different climate. They are also highly aware that they will be asked to talk about their experiences. Might all of this provoke some new sensations, thoughts, or emotions? I feel quite sure it would in me. It's well known that when one expects (or needs) to find a pattern, one is very likely to "find" it even if it isn't actually there—recall our familiar friend Orion.

After a proving, the analysts are surely highly motivated to discover something; in fact it would essentially be unacceptable *not* to find motifs, symptoms, an emergent personality or a characteristic trauma "in" the remedy. The organizers and attendees call this event a proving. But how confident should we be about our knowledge of the new remedy substance? Confident enough to call it a medicine and use it in practice?

There are dream provings, in which people put the remedy vial under their pillow one night; the contents of their dreams are taken as therapeutic indications for the remedy. There are meditation provings, in which a small group, or even just one person, sits with the remedy and attempts to let their intuition inform them of the conditions it is capable of healing.

Are people in these situations actually experiencing the remedy, though they have not ingested or touched it? The answer can only be: maybe? Both the remedies and human consciousness are far more subtle than standard chemistry and incompletely understood. Intuition is a real capacity of humans (though perhaps some of us tend to be too eager to call our thoughts by that name). The critical point is, we have no way of knowing what has come from the remedy, what from coincidence, what from imagination.

Many years ago, out of curiosity, I slept with a remedy vial in my hand. It was an interesting new partially-proved substance. The truth is, that night I had an extremely intense and unusual dream. I have had no other like it, before or since. But does it follow that I should analyze that dream, and apply *my* interpretation of *my* dream to the injury, disease, or psyche of other people? To me that seems more an act of ego than of science. Since I knew what the substance was, could the peculiar images of my dream have been partly due to the power of suggestion?

Are the new ways of proving and using the remedies true innovations, or are they distractions which lead our thinking astray? Do they clarify the process, or confuse it? Are they progressive, or irresponsible?

Here is a curious thing: almost all of the homeopaths conducting these provings will profess deep admiration for Hahnemann and the rational medical system he created; yet how very far some of these practices are from his exacting precision. What would he say today, faced with the disintegration of classical homeopathy in some schools and practices? For an answer to that question, we have only to look back at his own scathing remarks about medicine based on speculation.

Do we still need the original principles of homeopathy today? Some say, rules made two hundred years ago are no longer relevant and we should be liberated from them. Others counter that the basic rules of practice are not based on opinion or preference, nor were they even invented by people; they are simply guidelines provided by nature itself. The harmlessness and efficacy of treatment still depend upon them, just as the rhythm of the tides still depends on the moon's gravity. It would be hard to debate the fact that if Hahnemann had been less scientific, if he had approached medicine as some of the modern methods do, homeopathy could never have taken shape as a viable practice. It would have disappeared two centuries ago.

Sometimes reframing a question, or placing it in a different context, can help us see it more clearly. For instance: is it still important for engineering and construction to be based on knowledge of materials, mathematics, and the laws of physics? Or are these just old fashioned notions we no longer need? Can we now build our bridges out of whatever material is most attractive, or cheapest? Is a striking aesthetic design enough to ensure it is durable and safe?

Or, to bring the question back to healthcare: If you should be in an accident and rushed to a hospital, how would you feel about the doctor choosing medications for you based on the color of the packaging, or on the symbolism of their chosen spiritual doctrine, instead of abiding by the protocols established to save lives?

Some believe that a homeopath's creativity and spontaneity should not be dampened by logic, and science is an unnecessary, intrusive constraint (or just boring). Some have simply never actually thought about the reasons that underlie the rules.

The word "classical" might give the impression of something outdated. But nothing could be further from the truth. It is classical homeopathy which hard science and clinical trials are validating. It's classical homeopaths you will find doing fundamental research and clinical trials, practicing complementary and palliative care in hospitals worldwide, developing agrohomeopathy, teaching in universities, daily increasing homeopathy's reach and its good reputation.

Classical does not mean a practice which is inflexible, or a practitioner who is uncreative or insensitive to the spiritual aspects of life and healing. It does not mean that homeopaths who uphold the principles of this holistic science are not open-minded or that they simply stick to tradition for its own sake. There have been major innovations in classical homeopathy, from people who are still at work today. Because they are built on a sound foundation, they have made informed practice more effective, and brought hope and healing even in deep and complicated cases. There is always room to learn more, to refine the art, to deepen the science. We are far from fully understanding the complexities of a human being, the potentials of the remedies, and the process that allows them to work together.

What classical *does* mean is that the well-being of the patient—today and for their whole future—is the highest priority. And this means, in turn, that a homeopath (like any practitioner) needs to have the humility to realize that their intuition, while it has a role to play in the process, is neither omniscient nor infallible; it may be colored by imagination in ways they aren't aware of. It cannot be the sole basis for making decisions which impact people's health. It must be balanced with reason and confirmed knowledge. This is the ideal in all kinds of medicine, and indeed any other important profession.

It benefits all to maintain a high standard of safety, consistency, and accountability in healthcare. This allows the current generation to again strengthen the practice for those who will follow. Classical homeopathy also fosters integration of the fine work of scientists of all eras, and collaboration across all borders. It is so easy to take for granted (and many in natural medicine do) how much of our comprehension of what we are, and of how we can heal, is built from the mainstream scientific understanding we have inherited.

By now you have a good sense of the most polarizing questions in modern homeopathy. Probably, one of these general approaches will appeal to you more than another, or be more in alignment with your own point of view. I hope you will now feel able to meet and talk with a homeopath and know with confidence whether their practice is what you are looking for. Don't hesitate to ask your questions!

# 12
# Eight cases

The following are cases I have worked with personally. I chose these particular stories because each illustrates something important about homeopathy. Names and some other details have been changed.

## *Thomas: a severe burn*

In rural Canada, the roar of gas-powered log splitting machines is an integral part of autumn. My neighbor Thomas rented a log splitter, towed it home with his truck, filled its gas tank, and spent the afternoon splitting firewood. He paused to rest; he was tired, and absentmindedly placed a bare hand on the steel motor casing and leaned his weight on it.

I have no idea what the temperature of that metal was, but the burn was appalling. It takes a long time for medical help to arrive out there. In the moments it took him to walk up the driveway and into the house, his palm and fingers were blazing red, excruciatingly painful, and huge blisters were forming. He seemed stunned by the intensity.

I had seen good results with homeopathy for minor burns, but I was afraid; I thought he could even lose his hand. I assessed his state as best I could. I dissolved a remedy in water and had him take a sip of it every few minutes. The blistering halted within about twenty minutes. Over the next hour, I alternated two remedies. The pain was still intense, but the blisters were receding. He chose to go home rather than to the hospital.

The following day, there was no sign of blistering. The redness was reduced, appearing only in patches. On the evening of the third day after the accident, there were pink patches, and the hand felt tired and sore—but the pain was completely gone. A week later, you would not have guessed from looking at Thomas's hand that anything had occurred.

Not every injury will respond so quickly or completely. We began within a few minutes, which undoubtedly made a big difference. But I include this case because it shows how astonishingly powerful the natural healing process can be. Even after years of using remedies, I would have had a hard time believing this story if someone had related it to me. I was inspired anew by Thomas's case.

### *Emily: anxiety, phobias, dysmennorhea, acne, and headaches*

At the age of thirteen, Emily's family had moved long-distance several times and she was having great difficulty feeling secure in her own life. Being in a public place brought on intense anxiety and nausea. She couldn't bear to go into a restaurant or store, even when accompanied by her mother. Small sounds in the night filled her with fright and dread. She was certain she heard people coming up the stairs in the dark, and hallucinated rats and spiders running over her bed.

Emily had a constant fear of becoming mortally ill. She had become significantly underweight, because although her mother carefully prepared every meal at home, Emily would hallucinate worms in the food and could not eat. She had severe pains with her menstrual periods, which were seven or eight days long and too frequent. She had acne on her face and other parts of her body. Emily came home from school (on the days when she could manage to go) with a headache. But many days, she stayed home.

Emily would immediately go to her room and lay in bed after school; the many stimulations of the day left her desperately wanting quiet and solitude. She needed the light on, but pulled the covers over her face and lay still. Nothing seemed to help at all.

It was clear that in this case a patient, gentle detangling process was needed, probably involving a sequence of remedies. The first one I chose did not change most of Emily's symptoms, but over several weeks the night fears and hallucinations gradually subsided.

After about eight weeks, Emily took a second remedy. This time, there was improvement in her sense of overstimulation and anxiety. She went to school more often; when she came home she would sometimes stay downstairs and eat dinner with the family. She even agreed to go into a restaurant with her mother one weekend. They ended up ordering the food to take out and ate in the car, but her mother was still delighted with this. During the same period of time, her acne worsened. Her periods continued to be painful and long.

Over the following year, Emily had two more remedies. With some ups and downs, there was continued improvement of her emotional symptoms and gradually her skin cleared almost completely. She still had cramps with her period, but only for one day instead of three, and they were not as severe. Her cycle normalized.

Her mother updated me recently: Emily has not missed a day of school in many months, and has gone from barely-passing grades to excelling in the most challenging classes her high school offers. She's learning photography in her spare time and participating in debate tournaments in her province's capital. She has a small circle of good friends, and enjoys shopping and hanging out with them at cafes, or watching movies together at home. Emily is somewhat anxious, but mostly excited, about her upcoming move to university in a distant city, where she plans to study journalism.

Emily's mother wept while telling me all of this. Illness isn't the province only of the sick individual. It impacts families very deeply. Her dedication and love, combined with the deep and gentle action of the remedies, transformed her daughter's life.

Emily's case illustrates beautifully the principle of the direction of cure. First, the dreadful subconscious fears—the deepest manifestations of the disturbance—began to resolve. Then her energy level improved; she could handle the stimulation of everyday life. During this time some physical symptoms intensified, and that was a good sign: we want the disturbance to move from a deep, vital level to a more superficial level. This is the natural order of healing: moving the disturbance outward, reclaiming health first in the most vital areas. In this way it can be released gradually, gently, and safely. Emily first become able to be herself and enjoy her life; over time, her physical complaints resolved as well.

## *Sophie: a child with emotional challenges*

Sophie attracted a lot of attention from the very beginning of her life. She was intelligent, pretty, and had exceptional artistic skill. Even as a young child she was quickly becoming an accomplished painter.

But relating to other people was very difficult for her. She seemed to be tone-deaf to people's emotions and accidentally hurt their feelings, leading to almost constant conflicts at school and at home. Sophie felt keenly that she didn't fit in anywhere. She was teased by other children, and openly disliked by some teachers because she seemed determined to be contrary. A vicious cycle was underway: she was bullied by peers, reprimanded by teachers, and became more and more angry and confused.

Though she sometimes seemed so insensitive to the feelings of others, she felt extremely vulnerable inside. Eventually Sophie rejected all relationships and became completely withdrawn, except for occasional outbursts of rage. At the end of one term, Sophie's mother was told she would not be allowed to return to school.

Sophie was enraged at her mother's suggestion that they seek the help of a therapist or doctor and shut down even more. Her mother was at the end of her rope, now compelled to home school and struggling to keep any peace at home. Sophie flatly refused to talk about her experience. The observations of parents are always important, but especially so in this case.

She had no significant physical symptoms, but the more subtle constitutional indications were useful. I noted clues like her food desires and aversions, details related to sleep, reactions to weather, and other indications. These things might seem trivial, but actually they provide valuable information about the way an organism is reacting to and processing its environment. Sometimes people are surprised to find, after taking a remedy, that habits or cravings of many years spontaneously change. Most important was the observation of her attitudes and behaviors.

Sophie took several remedies over the course of two years. The first really good sign came after the second remedy: for the first time since infancy, she developed a rash on her arms and legs. It itched severely, but I strongly suggested the parents not suppress it with creams or prescriptions. The disturbance was moving outward: this was good progress. Preventing that expression in the skin could have halted her healing, confused her symptoms, or and even intensified her emotional suffering.

She also started having vivid dreams, and with a new openness, was willing to describe them to her mother. The persistent emotional themes in the dreams gave some very helpful insights.

Another milestone, after the next remedy, was the new ability she acquired to respect boundaries—her own, as well as those of other people. She could feel frustrated or hurt without immediately lashing out or shutting down. She could recognize the moments when she needed some breathing space, and found activities that helped her relax. Sophie took up music. Practicing every day seemed to help her stabilize. She made valiant efforts to face her own inner conflicts, and was rewarded by a new sense of self-confidence. For the first time in many years, she began to show a sense of humor.

A unique individual, Sophie will always be different from her peers. But she has now come to see this in a positive light, rather than suffering over it. Her case shows the importance of healing the inner distress, rather than suppressing it.

Her story could have gone very differently. In kindergarten her teachers were already suggesting Sophie wouldn't be able to manage in a regular school. By the second grade her parents were being pressured by school administrators and the extended family to give Sophie medications which would control her behavior. But they were concerned about where that would lead and how it would impact her health. They believed that there must be a better way. It required some sacrifice, especially on her mother's part: home schooling this extremely bright, intense, oppositional girl through the middle school years felt next to impossible.

But Sophie went back to school, and then to a prestigious university. Today she is a thriving artist with well-rooted confidence, strong relationships and a good life ahead of her. I love the way this case reminds us that homeopathy is not about changing our personalities or making us more "normal." It's about evolving into our own best, most unique selves and feeling more freedom in our lives. A lot of faith in the healing process was needed in this case; it has been well rewarded.

## *Andrew: food poisoning*

While traveling in Central America, Andrew, a ten year old boy, became very sick after eating in a restaurant. His parents suspect he was poisoned by the water; they had beer instead of water and didn't get sick.

Though the weather was very warm, Andrew was chilled and shivering. He had a frightened look and couldn't stay in bed, but paced back and forth, getting upset if his mother tried to leave the room. He had diarrhea, then began to throw up while having diarrhea. He wanted water, but would take only tiny sips.

This case was relatively simple. Andrew had one dose of a remedy at about 10:15 p.m. A few minutes later, his body made one more big effort and he threw up again. Then he began to relax. By 10:40, it was all over: the nausea was gone, the agitation was gone, his temperature was normal. He was weak and shaky from the event, but relieved and even cheerful. He slept soundly and was well the next morning.

Andrew's case is one which could have easily and safely been treated by a well-informed parent. His family traveled with an acute care remedy kit and we were able to work out what he needed over the phone.

## *Rachel: Chronic Fatigue Syndrome and autoimmune disease*

This case is full of complexity. This woman's health problems developed over many years. Chronic fatigue is notoriously hard to handle with conventional medicine. Symptoms vary greatly between individuals, and often a physiological cause isn't evident. But those individualized symptoms that may frustrate a doctor are very useful to a homeopath. Rachel didn't find homeopathy till she was in her forties, and years of trying different approaches had created a confusion of symptoms. But her commitment to regenerating her damaged immune system was strong.

Her health problems had begun in childhood, following traumatic events, amplified by the fact that there were no reliable adults to whom she could turn. The first phase of her healing through homeopathy brought much self-discovery. As the emotional problems began to resolve, a series of physical challenges presented, including the reappearance of old symptoms which had been suppressed but not cured in her past. In time, things she had experienced in early childhood and had completely forgotten about, such as nosebleeds, began to return. She even found she had gone back to sleeping in the posture she had preferred as a young child.

Rachel has not had an easy time working through old symptoms. Some have been very uncomfortable. What keeps her going is the knowledge that she's strengthening her system in the deepest way possible. She still doesn't have as much vitality as she would like; one way we know that is that she still doesn't get flus or colds with robust fevers. When the immune system doesn't have enough energy, it can't react against common pathogens. We look forward to the day when she raises a high temperature.

Sometimes the remedies can begin by lightening the emotional burden, and this sets free some energy. This in turn allows the exhausted body to recuperate. It's as if the body's systems begin to remember how to function with ease. Faith in the process grows, and a positive feedback cycle begins. There have been many changes over four years of working with Rachel, and her assessment now is that she's about 80% improved. When discouraged, she thinks about the condition she'd be in if she had chosen to use conventional medications instead and continually suppressed her immune system instead of regenerating it. Most importantly, she has the energy to enjoy things again—and she has hope. We continue.

## *Loki: a traumatized dog*

A friend asked me if I could help her dog. I'm not a veterinarian, but she wanted an alternative to conventional veterinary treatment for his trauma and I agreed to try.

She had adopted Loki as an adult dog. The only history we knew was that he had been attacked by a pack of other dogs. He was badly injured, and the owners opted to surrender him to a shelter.

His symptoms? He didn't have much in the way of physical symptoms. His demeanor was aloof; he wasn't friendly or affectionate. He liked to go outdoors, but definitely not on cold windy days. My friend also noted he was extremely sensitive to noises, especially loud, sudden sounds. And at a certain time every day, as the sun was going down, Loki would suddenly become terribly afraid. His behavior was what we would recognize in a human as a panic attack. He trembled, and paced the floor in great restlessness, eyes wide and full of fear.

Loki only had one dose, of a relatively high potency. His demeanor began to change right away. A few days later, my friend texted me about the transformation. For the first time since she had adopted him, he had relaxed. His anxiety attacks stopped, and he started to seek attention and to play. He went from traumatized "rescue" to affectionate pet within a week. Months later, he relapsed when his household went through some stressful changes. The indications were the same as before, and a second dose quickly cleared them.

Fortunately Loki was showing clear signs, and his human was observant. It always makes me sad to read stories of pets considered hopelessly traumatized, aggressive, or depressed; in so many cases, they could make good progress with homeopathic care. There are homeopathic veterinarians, but it can be hard to find one near you. The Academy of Veterinary Homeopathy website includes a directory.

## *A cucumber plant with bacterial wilt*

For a number of years now I've relied almost entirely on homeopathy for problems in my garden. There's a lot of experimentation involved. Plants' symptoms don't always easily correlate to human symptoms. But sometimes they do: for example, a combination of heat, dryness, and need for excessive amounts of water lead straight to one common remedy. A nutrient deficiency can be addressed in the plant, so the crop can be saved, while amending the soil would not solve the problem till the following year. Sometimes I miss the mark; but sometimes I get great results. It's a learning process.

One summer I was dismayed to find a cucumber plant, which had been thriving, with a limp branch. It was clearly bacterial wilt, which I knew is considered incurable. One is advised to quickly remove the whole plant and carefully dispose of it, keeping it away from one's soil and compost. But it's an infection, I thought; why not at least try to treat it homeopathically? After searching through some articles and repertories, I chose a remedy. I dissolved it in water in a spray bottle and gave the main stem of the plant a couple of good sprays—no need to try to spray everywhere; the minimum dose is all that's needed. I sprayed a little on the neighboring plants too, since they had almost certainly been infected.

The next day I found the one wilted limb shriveled and dry. The rest of the plant looked better than ever, healthy, green, energetic. I was in a rush and didn't even stop to remove the damaged part. I meant to come back and do it later in the day... but forgot.

I never did get around to cutting that dead branch off. There was no further sign of the disease in that plant or any other, even though all were undoubtedly exposed to the bacteria. A point to note in this case is that the remedy not only cured the sick plant; it preemptively "cured" the other plants' susceptibility to the infection.

### *Heartnut trees consumed by caterpillars*

Last year I saw a caterpillar I'd never noticed in the region before. More accurately, I saw hundreds of them, all over some young heartnut trees I was growing in planters. I did a little research and learned that this was a recently arrived invasive species. The leaves which they had already reached were eaten away completely, nothing remaining but their lacy skeletons.

Agrohomeopathy does not kill insects, or slugs, or even bacteria. It stimulates the plant to become resistant to the pest or disease, a process which takes plant breeders many generations to accomplish. It amounts to an extremely accelerated evolutionary adaptation, just as the right remedy allowed Emily to become comfortable with crowds and noise, and Andrew to rapidly overcome food poisoning. I treated my heartnut trees with a classic remedy for caterpillar infestation.

When I made it back out there the next day, the caterpillars had gone. It was like finding a meal half-eaten, abandoned, on a table: they had simply walked away. It was almost autumn, and they didn't return. I'm now curious to see whether they will be here next year; and if they are, will they react differently to the trees I treated? Do these trees now have more immunity to that pest?

This is one of the most exciting prospects of homeopathic care, whether in plants, animals, or humans: over generations, better immunity, adaptability, and resilience can be built. As living organisms, plants are subject to the laws of epigenetics too. When those trees mature, will their seedlings have greater natural resistance to caterpillars? Farmers, gardeners and seed saving enthusiasts have strengthened the genetics of plants for many thousands of years. It's reasonable to surmise that homeopathy can be of service in giving crops greater natural resistance to challenges.

Imagine the impact that homeopathy could have on agriculture and forestry: strengthening immunity, healing disease, creating more resilience to extreme climate conditions, halting blights that threaten whole crops (or even species) and the livelihoods of millions of people, and even rehabilitating damaged soils. It is already being done, in many locations on six continents, and expanding exponentially as people see the benefits unfold before their eyes. These projects need and deserve resources, attention, oversight, and more organized cooperative networks.

# 13
# Food for thought

I had been living in a remote area for years when I drove one morning to the nearest moderate-sized town and checked in at the emergency room of the hospital. Around forty people spent the day in that waiting room (it's open limited hours). One striking thing from that day: not a single person in the ER waiting room was having a medical emergency. We were all there because there are so few doctors in our province that a quarter of its residents have no family healthcare practitioner. The urgent care, walk-in clinics are few and far between, most are open just six or eight hours each week and often must turn people away.

When I was young and studied emergency medicine, a shift in the ER meant seeing people in desperate condition. I saw that again at those times when life is punctuated by sudden need. But here, at the day-to-day level of a deeply dysfunctional medical system, the ER is the last resort of the unserved.

Two people in the waiting room (one of them was me) needed diagnostic testing and had no doctor to request it from. Every other case could probably have been treated effectively with safe, simple care: healing foods, herbs, acupuncture, homeopathy, elementary bodywork such as a few acupressure points. In many cases all that was needed was some nourishing food, a little loving attention, and rest.

Certainly those would have served the several young children better than a long day being propped up, hushed, scolded, and bribed with sugary treats in a cold, damp, cheerless room full of people staring at their phones. Never underestimate the healing power for a child of a cozy blanket, a heartfelt smile, and a good story. Or the power of humanity's traditional medicines in knowledgeable hands.

How tragic that basic personal and family healthcare is disappearing. How wasteful that those people spent their day waiting for unnecessary immunity-degrading drugs. How disgraceful that their lifelong tax burdens are rewarded with such paucity. How onerous practicing medicine must feel, given that doctors decline to stay and work here despite automatic prestige and bountiful financial reward. How great the need to renew a basic ethos of caring for ourselves and each other; how good it would be to see less fear regarding sickness.

Being a willing participant in the natural healing process is a deeply rewarding undertaking which has been almost entirely abandoned by millions of people, in the name of progress. A profound, authentic optimism arises when we experience significant sickness healing naturally; the glow of well being growing in oneself is a unique and precious feeling. Yet many—probably most—modern people, at least in North America, have never in their lives had that experience. In its place we usually have uninformed and unquestioning patienthood and the confused, meaning-deprived sensations of a drugged organism.

Time and again I've seen people submitting to treatments which they *know* are making their health worse, or driving devastating "side" effects (in other words, iatrogenic sydromes) because they were told to do it by a doctor and they assume they have no choice. I'm sure you've seen that too. What a shame they are not encouraged to seek appropriate complementary or alternative care. Even simple questions are often discouraged.

I left the hospital after waiting for seven hours, never having made it into the back room. But the day inspired this epilogue: an appeal to troubled communities. Let's lift ourselves out of the rote routine of helpless habit; bring some engagement and hope into our hearts; open our minds with curiosity. Why not become active participants in our own lives and learn about our options?

Traditionally, it was understood everywhere (and in many places it still is) that the health of individuals is never separate from harmony in societies or from the larger ecosystem of life on Earth. The harsh consequences of forsaking this truth are evident all around us, at every scale. Human decisions have damaged not only our own health but the whole biosphere.

The value of homeopathic healthcare extends far beyond the borders of medicine. As a way of seeing ourselves and others, it can help heal families, communities, and societies. It offers us a new view of humanity: each of us a unique individual with the potential to contribute a particular good in the world. It fosters tolerance and optimism—a potent remedy for our anxious, fractured cultures.

In our own lives, homeopathy teaches us that illness is not an enemy to be viewed with aggression and fear. To view our sickness that way is to view our selves, and life itself, that way. Natural medicine invites us to know more deeply what we are. It can teach us, if we're willing, in ways that no other experience can, about being, and becoming. When we respect the gift of life we are being given, we will be on the way to realizing that it does not serve anyone to see illness and medicine in terms of warfare, terror, and despair.

We live in a time of momentous global changes, and important choices are available to us. Healthcare is poised to enter a new era: safer, more affordable, more humane, more effective, more optimistic, more individualized, more sustainable. If we embrace the potential of natural medicines, study and refine them intelligently—while refining conventional medicine alongside—we can begin to reverse the widespread decline in immunity, hope, and quality of life. We can move away from needlessly poisoning our environment and crushing our economies with profit-hungry systems that drive our culture toward collapse. Willingly evolving our understanding of health and disease is a first and vital step for our own well-being, for the coming generations, and even for our planet.

# References


1. WHO Global Report on Traditional and Complementary Medicine 2019, *World Health Organization,* 2019.

2. "Homeopathy in Europe: used, appreciated and well-known," *European Commission on Homeopathic and Anthroposophic Medicinal Products,* April 10, 2023.

3. Jamie Ducharme, "More that 70% of Americans Feel Failed by the Health Care System," *Time,* May 16 2023.

4. Sylvie Piché, "Survey on Homeopathy awareness and usage in Canada: 10.3 million Canadians used homeopathy in 2022, Cision, June 19, 2023.

5. Manjiri Kanhere, "Homeopathy Product Market Report 2025 (Global Edition)", *Cognitive Market Research (*March 2025).

6. "Survey results reveal the challenges experienced by family doctors," *Canadian Institute for Health Information,* accessed January 2025.

7. Antonei B. Csoka and Moshe Szyf, "Epigenetic side effects of common pharmaceuticals: a potential new field in medicine and pharmacology," *Medical Hypotheses,* 73 no.5 (November 2009):770-780.

8. "The Problem of Pharmaceutical Pollution," *European Environment Bureau,* accessed October 2024.

9. Suong-Mai Vu Ngoc et al., "COVID-19 and environmental health: A systematic analysis for the global burden of biomedical waste by this epidemic," *Case Studies in Chemical and Environmental Engineering,* 6, December 2022.

10. Gabrielle Masson, "Drug Development Cost Pharma $2.2B per asset in 2024 as GLP1s drive financial return: Deloitte," *Fierce Biotech,* March 25, 2025.

11. Aylin Sertkaya et al., "Costs of Drug Development and Research and Development Intensity in the US, 2000-2018," *JAMA Network Open,* June 28, 2024.

12. Mike Cummings, "Novel study quantifies immense economic costs of mental illness in the U.S.," *YaleNews,* April 22, 2024.

13. Jamie Ducharme, "America Has Reached Peak Therapy. Why Is Our Mental Health Getting Worse?,"*Time,* August 30, 2023.

14. Todd Cooney, "Understanding the role of homeopathy in epidemics," *Innovative Veterinary Care,* accessed May 2025.

15. Richard Haehl, *Samuel Hahnemann: His Life & Work Volume I,* 177-179, B. Jain Publishers Ltd., 2016.

16. Michael Emmans Dean, "Homeopathy and 'The Progress of Science,'" *History of Science,* 39: 225-283.

17. Haehl, 178-179.

18. Jerry Kantor, *Sane Asylums: The Success of Homeopathy Before Psychiatry Lost Its Mind,* Healing Arts Press, 2022.

19. Richard Hammerschlag et al., "Biofield physiology: a framework for an emerging discipline," *Global Advantages in Integrative Medicine and Health* 4 (Suppl) (November 1, 2015):35-41. https://doi.org/10.7453/gahmj.2015.015.suppl

20. Haiying Wang et al., "Bioelectric Fields as Signalling Currents of Life," *Radiation Medicine and Protection,* 6 no.2 (April 2025): 112-118.

21. Tianjun Liu, "The Scientific Hypothesis of an 'energy system' in the Human Body," *Journal of Traditional Chinese Medical Sciences,* 5 no.1 (January 2018): 29-24.

22. Veronica Salib, "Can Pharmaceutical Companies Ethically Sponsor Medical Education?", *Informa* (September 19, 2023).

23. Michael A. Steinman and Robert B. Baron, "Is continuing medical education a drug-promotion tool? YES," *College of Family Physicians* 53 no.10 (October, 2007):1650-1653.

24. Hannah Fresques, "Doctors Prescribe More of a Drug If They Receive Money from a Pharma Company Tied To It," *ProPublica* (December 20, 2019).

25. Edward J. Calabrese, "Hormesis and medicine," *British Journal of Clinical Pharmacology* 66 no. 5 (July 25, 2008):594-617.

26. "Compendium of Homeopathic Research," *Americans for Homeopathy Choice,* accessed January 2025.

27. *Homeopathy Research Institute,* accessed January 2025.

28. *Initiative to Promote Research in Homeopathy,* accessed January 2025.

29. Camelia Berghian-Grosan et al., "Ultra-high Dilution Analysis: Exploring the Effects of Potentization by Electron Microscopy, Raman Spectroscopy, and Deep Learning, *Journal of Molecular Liquids,* 401 (May 2024).

30. Gerald H. Pollack, *The Fourth Phase of Water,* Ebner and Sons Publishers, 2013.

31. Vladimir Voeikov and Konstantin Korotkov, "The Emerging Science of Water," *International Union of Medical and Applied Bioelectrography,* January 10, 2018.

32. Steven Cartwright, "Physico-chemical properties of succussed high dilutions," *hri-research.org,* accessed January 2025.

33. Steven Cartwright, "Investigating photon emissions from homeopathic potencies," *International Journal of High Dilution Research,* 24 no.1 (February 12, 2024):10-11.

34. George Vithoulkas and Camelia Berghian-Grosan, "The Spin of Electrons and the Proof for the Action of Homeopathic Remedies," *Journal of Medicine and Life,* 13 no.3 (July-September 2020):278-282.

35. Katarina Zimmer, "'Social' Mitochondria, Whispering Between Cells, Influence Health," *Quanta,* July 6, 2021.

36. Olli Matilainen et al., "Mitochondria and Epigenetics—Crosstalk in Homeostasis and Stress," *Trends in Cell Biology* 27 no.6 (June 2017):453-563.

37. Kelley S. Joubert et al., "A Review of Preclinical Research on the Effects of Photodynamic Therapy and Homeopathic Medicine on Cancer Cells," *Alternative Therapies in Health and Medicine* 27 no. 6 (November 2021):40-50.

38. Marc Henry, "The Physics and Chemistry of High-Dilutions," *Homeopathy and You* 5 no. 2(March 2019).

39. Lionel R. Milgrom, "Towards a New Model of the Homeopathic Process Based on Quantum Field Theory, *Forschende Komplementärmedizin / Research in Complementary Medicine* 13 no. 3 (July 2006):174-183.

40. Antonio Manzalini and Bruno Galleazi, "Explaining Homeopathy with Quantum Electrodynamics, Homeopathy 108 no. 3 (August 2019):169-176.

*An extended bibliography is available at*
***https://www.smratliff.com/homeopathy-rising***

# Index

Academy of Veterinary Homeopathy 128
acupuncture 52, 62, 87, 134
agrohomeopathy 81, 81, 112, 130
allopathic medicine 13
Americans for Homeopathy Choice 140
animals 11, 79
antibiotics 4, 29, 32, 78, 80
apophenia 109
apprenticeship 92

biological systems 11, 55
biology 31, 50, 55, 61, 66, 67, 68

Canada 115, 138
cancer 23, 24, 68, 79
combination remedies 34, 88, 101, 102, 128
contrary medicine 12, 13

diet 21, 31, 41, 54, 58, 70
direction of cure 38, 119
DNA 26, 68

Earth 3, 3–147, 4, 4–147, 74, 95, 136
energy fields, human 51, 52, 65, 67, 69
epidemics 4, 35, 40, 41
epigenetics 31, 58, 68, 70, 131
Europe 3, 40, 44

frequency 47, 57, 101

genetic expression 31, 32
genetics, study of 43
gravity 74, 111

Hahnemann, Samuel 9, 42, 44, 55, 58, 59, 60, 70, 71, 74, 75, 106, 107, 110, 111, 139

herbs, herbal medicine 21-23, 15, 39, 54, 55, 88, 92, 104, 134
Homeopathy Research Institute 140

imagination *see* intuition
immunity, immune system 4, 22, 24, 31, 32, 34, 41, 45, 47-49, 58, 125, 126, 131, 134, 137
infection, infectious disease 4, 32, 40, 42, 46, 48, 78-80, 85, 105, 129, 130
intuition 99, 100, 109, 113

Kingdom Method 98

law of similars 55, 57, 94

meditation 109
mental illness 37, 42, 139
minimum dose 59, 103, 104, 129
mitochondria 67, 68
moon 111, 143

North America 22, 29, 44, 73, 91, 135

*Organon of the Medical Art* 9
Orion 99, 109

palliative care 112
Periodic Table 95, 96
placebo 7, 40, 77-79, 81, 107, 110
pluralism 102, 105
pregnancy 85
proving 55, 106, 107, 108, 110
provings, homeopathic 106–147
pseudoskeptics 1, 72
psychotherapy 35, 37, 38

quantum physics 60, 68

research 5, 7, 7–147, 1, 5, 51, 52, 61, 61–147, 62, 63, 64, 69, 71, 112, 130, 140, 143

Research In Homeopathy 62
resonance 47, 101
Roman Catholic Church 49

Sensation Method 94, 97, 98
side effects 4, 15, 28, 55, 102, 138
similar medicine 11, 39, 54, 55, 57, 58, 94
similimum, defined 58
solvatochromic dyes 67
soul 50, 98
Staphysagria 34
Strasbourg University 68
Sulphur 34
suppression 12, 22, 30, 35, 46, 48, 58, 113, 122, 123, 125
susceptibility 24, 25, 130

*The Chronic Diseases* 43
trauma 4, 30, 37, 38, 41, 43, 70
tuning fork 47, 101

unicist homeopathy 57
University of Johannesburg 68

veterinarians, homeopathic 80, 128
vital force 11, 47, 48, 49, 51, 52, 57, 58, 102, 105

water 33, 46, 54, 64, 66, 69, 116, 124, 128, 130
World Health Organization 2, 138

# Image credits

Cover image: Song_about_summer via Adobe Stock

Frontispiece: "Ultra-high dilutions analysis: Exploring the effects of potentization by electron microscopy, Raman spectroscopy, and deep learning," Camelia Berghian-Grosan, Sahin Isik, Alin Sebastan Porav, Ilknur Dag, Kursad Osman Ay, and George Vithoulkas, *Journal of Molecular Liquids* 401 (May 2024). Used by permission. Creative Commons license number 5990140508551.

Back cover image: "Datura Stramonium," Peter Esser, *Die Giftpflanzen Deutschlands,* 1910. Public domain.

# Acknowledgements

I wish to express my deepest respect and gratitude to Dr. Hahnemann, and to all who have furthered true homeopathy. For their insights and support in the creation of this book, I extend my thanks to Azza elBakry, Sarah Martin, and Nancy Tam.

# About the author

S. Marjorie Ratliff integrates classical homeopathy with holistic nutrition and other healing arts via online consultations, and offers an online course about holistic strategies for preventing and healing cancer. She is an author, an organic master gardener, and an educator. To learn more, please visit *smratliff.com*.

www.ingramcontent.com/pod-product-compliance
Lightning Source LLC
La Vergne TN
LVHW100319210926
848480LV00003B/1181
*9781069176523*